AF863727

ECG

A Practical Guide to the ECG Interpretation in Hospital and General Practice

H. Löllgen (MD)

Layout and art work:

STUDIO Z
Corporate Communication
Ockenheimer Chaussee 5
D-6530 Bingen

All rights reserved.
No part of this publication may be reproduced or copied in any form or by any means – graphic, electronic or mechanical including photo copying, recording, taping, or information on retrieval systems – without permission of the publisher.

Contents

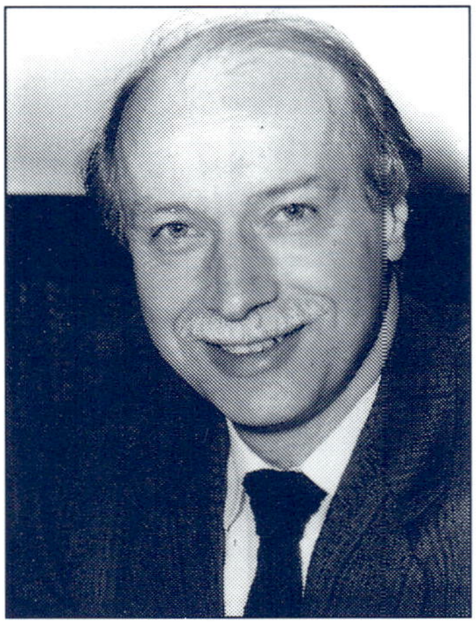

Herbert Löllgen (MD)
Professor of Medicine (Cardiology)
Ruhr-University of Bochum
Germany

Curriculum vitae

Specialist in internal medicine:
Medical Clinic, University Hospital Cologne (Prof. Gross)
University Hospital Mainz, Medical Clinic II
(Prof. Schölmerich)

Physiology, pneumology:
Bethanien Hospital, Moers (Prof. Worth)

Cardiology:
University Hospital Mainz, Medical Clinic II
(Prof. Schölmerich, Prof. Just)

Traineeship:
August-Krogh Institute, Copenhagen (Prof. Saltin)
Senior registrar of University Hospital Freiburg, Medical Clinic III (Cardiology, Prof. Just)
Head of Medical Clinic, Cardiology
Vincenz Hospital, Limburg (1983)
Head of Medical Clinic, Cardiology
Remscheid Hospital (1986)
Academic Hospital, Ruhr-University, Bochum

Scientific interests:
Cardiopulmonary functional diagnostics, emergency medicine, rhythm disturbances, aero-space medicine

Preface

This manual was originally issued as a brochure to explain a new ECG calculator. Both the ECG calculator and the brochure have been met with encouraging interest. After several reprints (in German), a more detailed manual was requested. The revised and enlarged edition contains additional definitions, examples and suggestions for interpretation. This book is meant to be neither an ECG manual nor a systematical course. It is a practical tool in the routine interpretation of the ECG.

Remscheid, May 1992

H. Löllgen

Use of the ECG Calculator

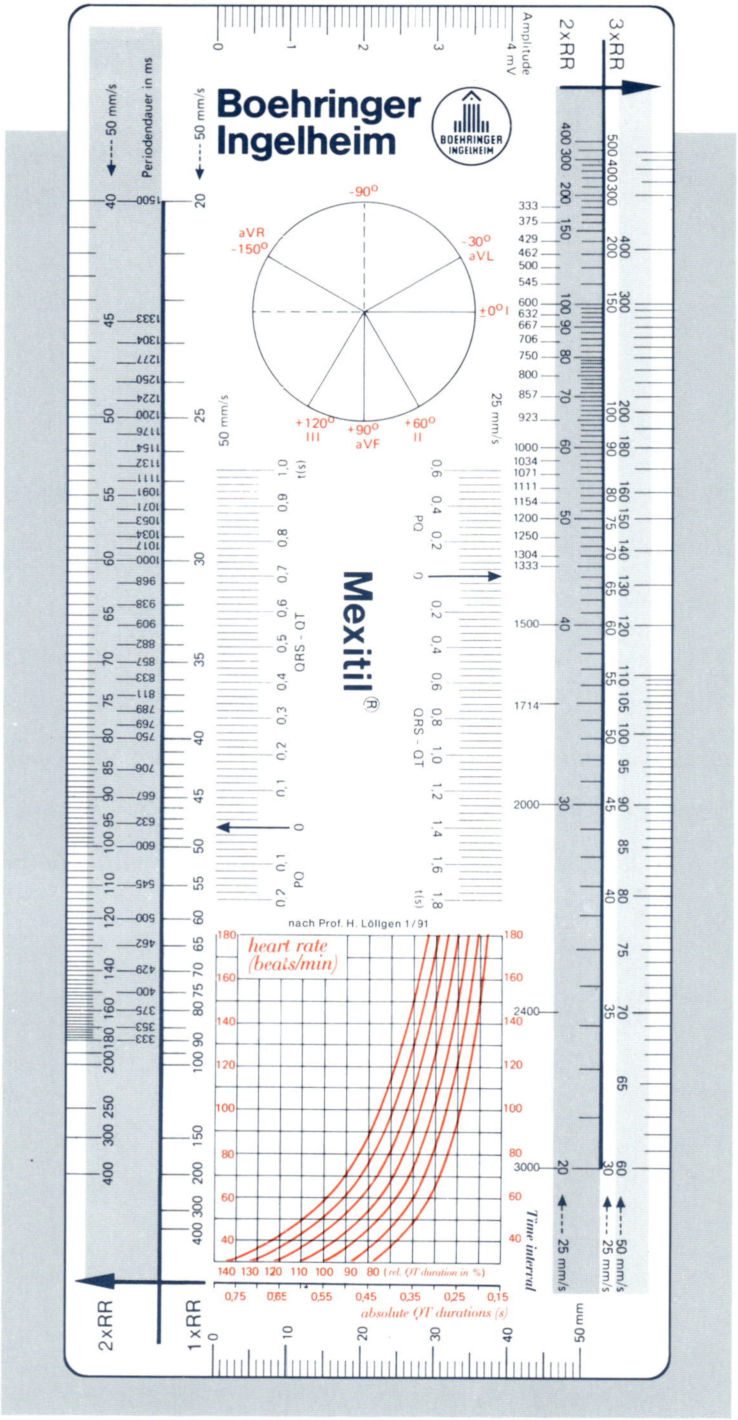

Use of the ECG Calculator

Heart rate

Calculation of heart rate: The scales on the edge give the heart rate for 3 and 2 cycles (3 RR intervals resp. 2 RR intervals) at a paper speed of 50 or 25 mm/s. The evaluation is shown in Fig. 1.

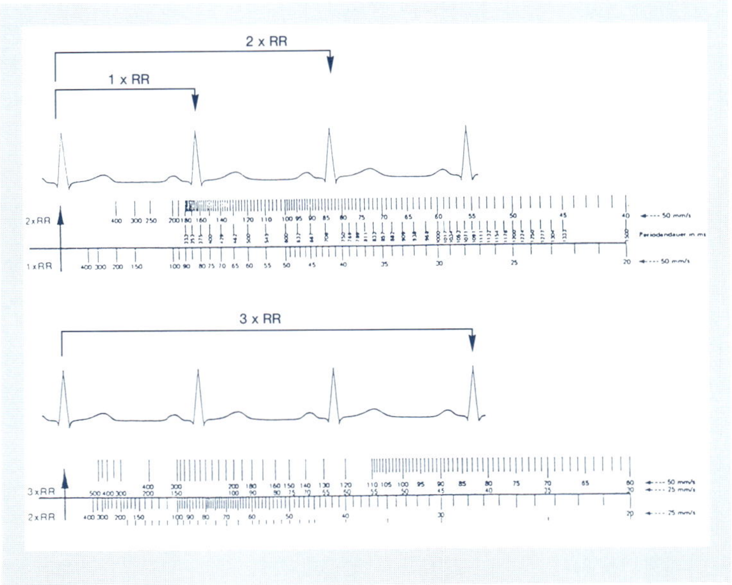

Fig. 1

Calculation of heart rate with the ECG calculator

The other edge of the calculator contains scales for the calculation of heart rate by 2 cycles or 1 cycle and the scale for the time interval at a paper speed of 50 mm/s.

Time interval
(RR interval)

Below the scale of heart rate (RR interval) the scales for time interval in milliseconds (ms) are given, according to the two paper speeds of 25 and 50 mm/s.

The time interval is reciprocal to heart rate. When analysing the pacemaker's rate, reference is usually made to the RR period. With the help of the two adjacent scales, RR period and pacing frequency are easily converted into each other.

From this scale (RR period) the sinus node recovery time can also be read off using a paper speed of **100** mm/s. On the scale "**2** x RR; **50** mm/s" the interval **1** x RR with a paper speed of **100** mm/s is to be measured. The reciprocal value can be taken as the sinus node recovery time in ms.

QT duration

The relative QT duration can be calculated by using the diagram in the middle of the calculator: take the absolute QT duration (beginning of QRS to the end of the T wave). The scale above the absolute QT duration refers to the lines of the relative QT duration in the diagram. The intercept of the absolute QT duration with heart rate (ordinate) gives the relative QT duration which can be read off between the curves.

The reading of the relative QT duration is illustrated in the following figure. Table 1 contains the corresponding absolute values.

Fig. 2

Calculation of the relative QT duration with the ECG calculator

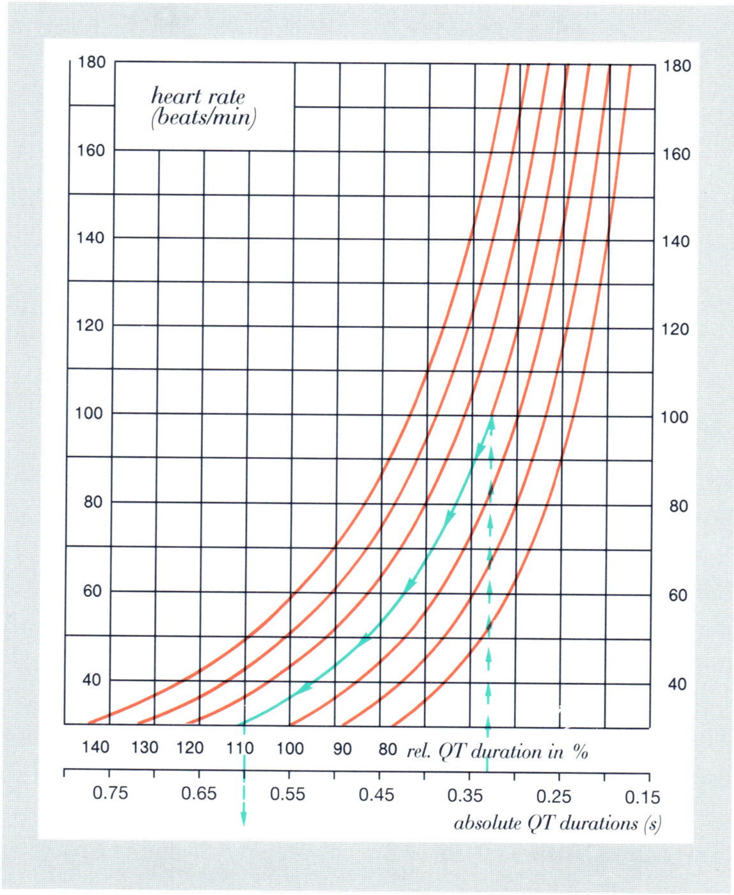

Example:
absolute QT duration = 0.32 s
heart rate = 100/min
relative QT duration = 110 %

heart rate	*men, children*	*women*	*upper limits men, children*	*upper limits women*
min $^{-1}$	*sec*	*sec*	*sec*	*sec*
40.0	0.449	0.461	0.491	0.503
43.0	0.438	0.450	0.479	0.491
46.0	0.426	0.438	0.466	0.478
48.0	0.420	0.432	0.460	0.471
50.0	0.414	0.425	0.453	0.464
52.0	0.407	0.418	0.445	0.456
54.5	0.400	0.411	0.438	0.449
57.0	0.393	0.404	0.430	0.441
60.0	0.386	0.396	0.422	0.432
63.0	0.378	0.388	0.413	0.423
66.5	0.370	0.380	0.404	0.414
70.5	0.361	0.371	0.395	0.405
75.0	0.352	0.362	0.384	0.394
80.0	0.342	0.352	0.374	0.384
86.0	0.332	0.341	0.363	0.372
92.5	0.321	0.330	0.351	0.360
100.0	0.310	0.318	0.338	0.347
109.0	0.297	0.305	0.325	0.333
120.0	0.283	0.291	0.310	0.317
133.0	0.268	0.276	0.294	0.301
150.0	0.252	0.258	0.275	0.282
172.0	0.234	0.240	0.255	0.262

Table 1

Reference values for QT related to heart rate

From: Essentials of Electrocardiography by R. Ashman and E. Hull, The Macmillan Company, New York, 1945.

Electrical axis

The inner field of the calculator gives the Cabrera circle for analysing the vector in the frontal plane (electrical axis)(Fig. 4 and Fig. 5). Next to the Cabrera circle two scales are shown for measuring the time intervals of the ECG (Fig. 3).

P wave	beginning of P	to end of P
PR interval (AV time)	beginning of P	to QRS complex
QRS complex	beginning of Q	to end of S wave
QT interval	beginning of Q	to end of T wave
ST segment	J point	to beginning of T wave
T wave	beginning of T	to end of T wave

The short edge of the calculator gives scales for measuring the amplitude of P, R, S and T at a calibration of 10 mm = 1 mV (Fig. 3).

Fig. 3

Scheme of the normal ECG for determination of amplitude and time intervals (modified by So)

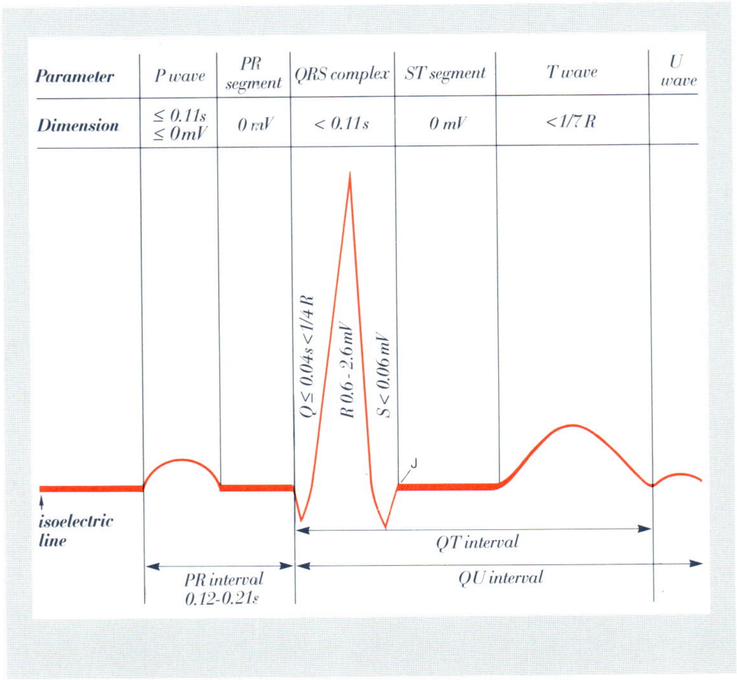

Diagnosis by the ECG

Diagnosis by the ECG

	Definitions
Sinus rhythm	Regular activation of atria and ventricles with constant PR interval
Bradycardia	Three or more consecutive impulses arising from the same pacemaker at a rate below the inherent rate of the pacemaker
Sinus bradycardia	Sinus rhythm at a rate under 60/min
Tachycardia	Three or more consecutive impulses from the same pacemaker at a rate exceeding 100/min
Sinus tachycardia	Sinus rhythm at a rate exceeding 100/min
Arrest	Cessation of electrical activity of the heart or part of it (sinus, ventricular)
Block	Delay or failure of impulse propagation
First degree AV block	PR interval above 0.20 s
Second degree AV block	Regular or irregular absence of the QRS complex following regular P waves. The PP interval remains constant
a) Mobitz I	Progressing lengthening of the PR interval until a QRS complex drops out (Wenckebach)
b) Mobitz II	Drop out of the QRS complex in regular intervals. The ratio of the absent QRS complexes to AV conduction may vary (2:1, 3:1, 3:2, 4:3 etc.). The PR interval remains constant
Third degree AV block	Complete dissociation of the activation of the atria and ventricles (no constant relation between P and R). The ventri-

cular rhythm may be the result of a higher located pacemaker (atrioventricular junction) (narrow QRS complex, heart rate 50-60/min) or a lower located impulse formation (ventricle) at a rate of 30-40/min and a widened QRS complex

SA block

Period with absent P waves lasting up to several seconds, ended by an activation of the ventricle by impulse formation either in the sinus node or the AV node (junctional rhythm). Occasionally also a ventricular escape rhythm can occur (widened QRS complex)

Escape beat

One or two consecutive impulses arising from the same pacemaker site as a result of undue delay in the formation or arrival of the dominant rhythm

Escape rhythm

Three or more consecutive escapes

Extrasystole

A premature impulse that shows a fixed relation to the preceding discharge of another pacemaker (atria, AV junction, ventricle)

Fibrillation

Rapid and irregular, disorganized electrical activity of the atria or ventricles. The ECG deflections of the fibrillating chamber change continuously in shape, duration and amplitude. In atrial fibrillation, the ventricular response is totally irregular. In ventricular fibrillation, QRS complexes can no longer be identified

Flutter

Rapid (>250/min) and regular electrical activity of the atria or ventricles, characterized in at least one lead by the absence of an isoelectric line in between the deflections of the fluttering chamber

Atrial tachycardia	Regular P waves (rate 160-220/min)
- with 1:1 conduction	Each P wave is followed by a QRS complex
- with AV block	Usually 2:1 block. Frequently a sign of digitalis overdosage
Atrial flutter	Regular P waves (rate 250-350/min). Sawtooth appearance, typically displayed in lead III. Usually associated with AV block (varying conduction ratio, 2:1 to 4:1), negative flutter waves in the inferior leads (III, aVF)
Atrial fibrillation	Absence of regular electrical activity of the atria. Irregular ventricular rate. The "isoelectric line" displays irregular oscillations of changing appearance. Fibrillation waves close to 350/min
Junctional rhythm	Regular activation of the atria associated with 1:1 conduction (rate 50-100/min). Negative P wave in II, III aVF. Short PR interval, the P wave frequently within the QRS complex or following it
Accelerated junctional rhythm	Junctional rhythm at a rate exceeding 100/min
Idioventricular	Regular (or slightly irregular) ventricular rhythm at a rate of 30-40/min. Widened, notched QRS complex, absence of preceeding P waves
Accelerated idioventricular rhythm	Automatic ectopic ventricular rhythm at a rate of 60-120/min
Ventricular fibrillation	Rapid irregular acitvation of the ventricles (= cardiac arrest)

Determination by the Cabrera circle

The lead with the largest QRS deflection points to the mean QRS axis (angle alpha) the lead with the smallest deflection (R = S) points to the lead perpendicular to it (Figs. 4 and 5).

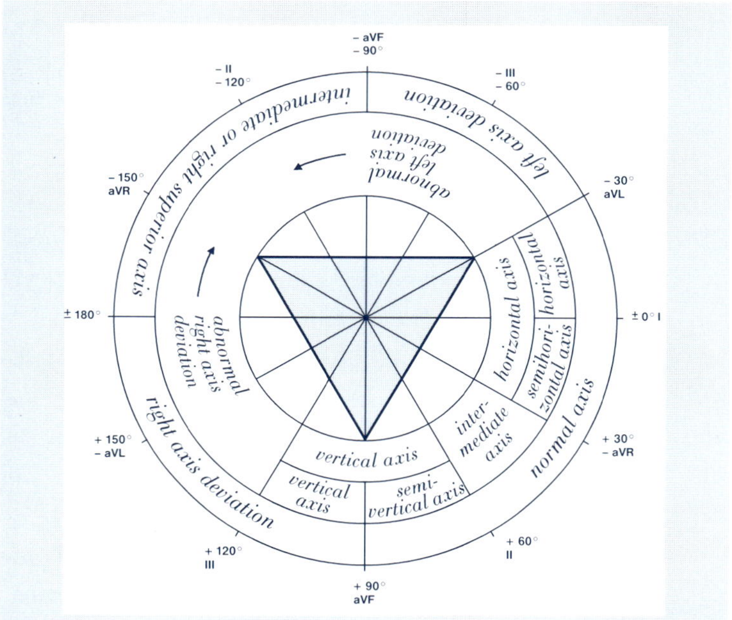

Marriot et al, Goldman et al 1982

Fig. 4

Cabrera circle for determination of the electrical axis. The mean vector in the frontal plane (limb leads) indicated by the highest R deflection. The angle between this vector and the horizontal line reflects the angle α

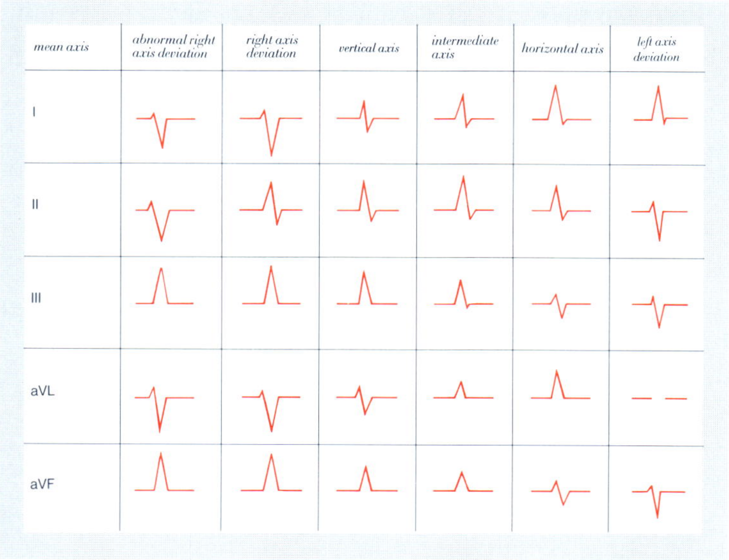

Fig. 5

Schematic presentation of R and S deflection at variable mean QRS axis

Selection of some criteria

Right ventricular hypertrophy

(Abnormal) right axis deviation

Example:
Page 66

Tall R waves in V_1 (>0.5 mV), R/S ratio in V_1 exceeding 1st ST segment depression in V_1 and inverted T, qR in V_1, beginning of intrinsicoid deflection exceeding 0.03 s in V_1, persistent S in V_5, V_6

Remember:

These criteria are found not infrequently in younger people without evidence of right ventricular strain.

The pattern of incomplete right bundle branch block (rSR) is often to be observed in young and physically fit people.

The above mentioned criteria suggest right ventricular hypertrophy. Interpretation should take place in a clinical context.

Left ventricular hyperthrophy

R wave in V_5 or V_6 greater than 27 mm, S in V_1 or V_2 + R in V_5 or V_6 greater than 35 mm (Sokolow-Lyon-Index)

Example:
Page 67

These are normal variants in young people of thin stature!

Onset of intrinsicoid deflection in V_1, V_1 exceeding 0.05 s

ST segment depression and/or T inversion in V_5, V_6

R in aVL greater than 1.3 mV, $R_1 + S_3$ greater than 2.6 mV

The stages of evolution of the ECG in acute infarction are shown in Fig. 6.

ECG stage		ECG changes
acute infarction (acute stage)	stage 1	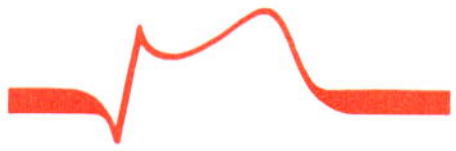
	intermediate stage	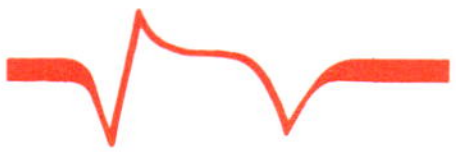
old infarction (chronic stage)	stage 2	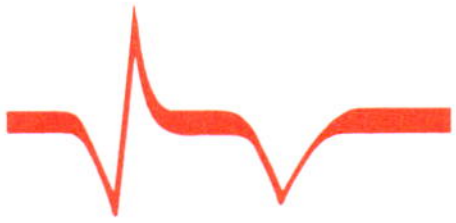
	stage 3	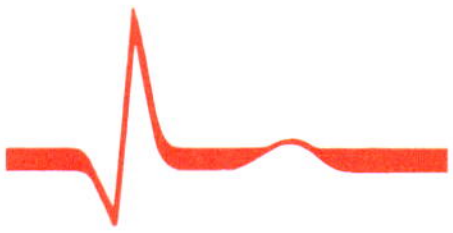

Fig. 6

Schematic presentation of the stages of evolution in acute infarction. Initially ST segment elevation, followed by development of a terminal negative T wave and a Q wave, finally a Q wave indicating the completion of the infarction

The infarction sites are classified by 4 localizations (Table 2, Fig. 7).

Localisation	**Typical change in lead**
Anterolateral	V_2-V_4 (V_5) (I)
Anteroseptal	I, (V_3), V_4-V_6 (aVL)
Inferior (diaphragmatical)	III, aVF, Nehb-D
Strictly posterior	V_2 (mirror image)

Combinations of different localizations are not unusual, e.g. anteroseptal extending to the lateral wall, inferior including the lateral wall or strictly posterior site (Figs. 8 and 9).

Occasionally, the absence of the septal Q ($Q_{I,\ aVL,\ V_6}$) is the only indication of an old anteroseptal infarction.

Table 2:

Localization of infarction

Term	**Coronary abnormality**	**Typical localization in the ECG**
Extended anterior infarction	proximal occluded left anterior descending artery (LAD)	V_2-V_5 I, II aVL
Anteroseptal infarction	occlusion of part of the peripheral LAD and its septal rami	V_1-V_3 (V_4)
Apical anterior infarction	occlusion of part of the peripheral LAD	V_3-V_4 (II)
Anterolateral infarction	Occlusion of part of the peripheral LAD and the ramus diagonalis	V_4 (V_3)-V_6 I, (II) VL
Inferolateral infarction	Occlusion of the ramus marginalis of the left coronary artery	V_5-V_6 (V_7) II-III aVF
Inferior (diaphragmatical) infarction	Occlusion of peripheral parts of the right coronary artery or the left ramus circumflexus	II, III aVF
Strictly posterior infarction	Occlusion of peripheral parts and branches of the left ramus circumflexus, especially of the ramus atrioventricularis	V_2 (V_1-V_3) reciprocal (II, III) (aVF)

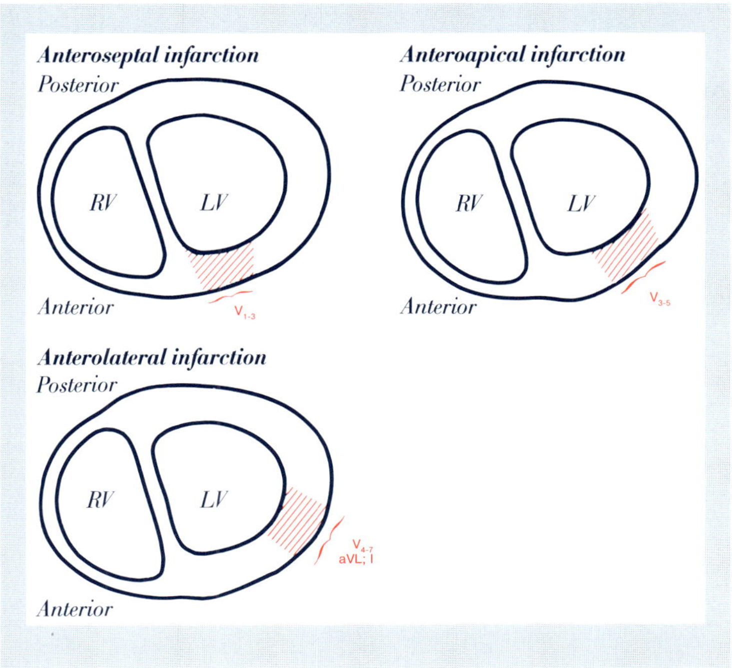

Fig. 7

Schematic presentation of the stages of anterior infarction in different localisation

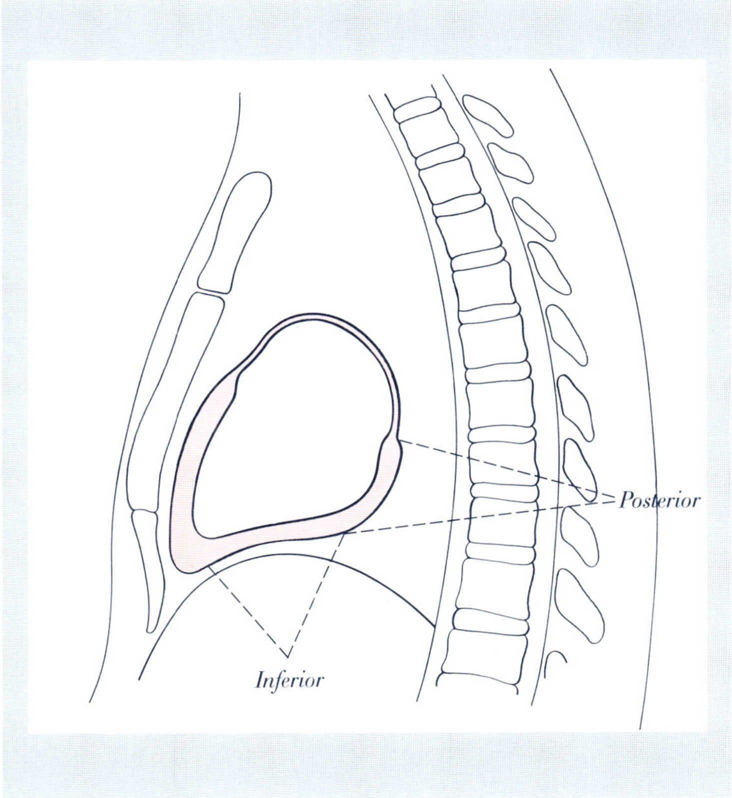

Fig. 8

Schematic presentation with differentiation between the inferior (or diaphragmatical) and posterior (or strictly posterior) localization. The posterior infarction is reflected inversely in the chest lead V_2

Abnormal Repolarisation

Repolarisation abnormalities vary in their appearance (Fig. 9). There is a large list of pathogenetic factors (Table 3).

Repolarisation abnormalities are not neccessarily due to ischaemia or "coronary" etiology, they have to be interpreted in the clinical context. The pathogenesis as shown in Table 2 has to be clarified in any case.

Table 3

Causes of abnormal repolarisation

1. Functional Causes

Example: Normal variant
sportsmen
"neurovegetative" related changes

2. Cardiac Causes

Mismatch of oxygen demand and oxygen supply (not identical with coronary heart disease)

2.1 Organic coronary sclerosis

2.2 Functional lack of perfusion
Hypertrophy, dilatation
Tachycardia
Anaemia
Hypoxia

2.3 Inflammatory heart diseases (pericarditis, myocarditis)

2.4 Primary myocardial diseases (congestive cardiomyopathy, hypertrophic (non-)obstructive cardiomyopathy, restrictive myocardial disorders)

3. Extracardiac disorders

Cerebral disorders (brain oedema, stroke)
Metabolic disorders
Intoxication
Electrolyte disturbances
Drugs (antineoplastic drugs, antiarrhythmic drugs, tricyclic antidepressants etc.)

Typical forms of abnormal repolarisation (by Heinecker). Downward coving ST segments are more likely to occur with digitalis therapy, downsloping ST segments are indicative of left ventricular hypertrophy. Always remember to interprete in the clinical context.

Fig. 9

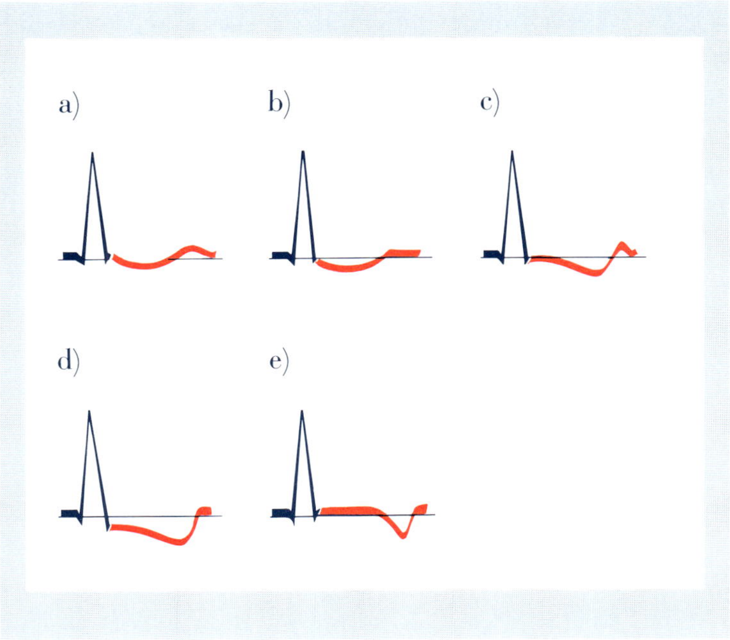

a) Downward coving ST segment depression with flattened T wave

b) Downward coving ST segment depression with isoelectric T wave

c) Upward convex ST segment depression, −/+ alternating T wave

d) Upward convex ST segment depression, preterminal negative T wave

e) Close T wave inversion or terminal negative T wave

Bradycardias

Definition

A rate below 60/min is called bradycardia

Remember:
Bradycardia is not always a sign of illness. Healthy people and sportsmen may have resting heart rates of as little as 35-40/min. Clinical signs and symptoms must be considered when interpreting.

Causes of bradycardia

Effect of physical endurance training in sportsmen

Vagal reactions

Hypothermia

Myxoedema and hypothyroidism

Drugs: digitalis, β-blockers, calcium channel blockers, (clonidine), α-methyldopa, tricyclic antidepressants

Uraemia, electrolyte disturbances

Disorders of the SA or AV node due to coronary heart disease, cardiomyopathy, myocarditis, cardiac surgery, congenitally, tumor

Idiopathic fibrosis (Lenègre's and Lev's disease)

Diagnosis

ECG at rest and holter monitoring

Atropine test (1-2 mg i.v.): Pathological: increase in heart rate of less than 90/min or less than 25 % of the starting rate

Exercise testing: Pathological: inadequate rise of heart rate (chronotropic incompetence) or fall in rate

Sinus node recovery time (SNRT): Stimulations in rates between 80 and 180/min over 30 s per period

The SNRT (in ms) is the time needed from the last stimulated P wave to the first spontaneous P wave

Pathological: Pause after stimulation exceeding 1500 ms (Seipel) or 1040 + 220 ms

The SNRT corrected for rate: 270 + 110 ms or 525 ms. Calculation: SNRT – mean RR period (n = 10) in ms

Carotid sinus massage: One sided massage of the region of the carotis sinus with the heart rate being observed: Table 4

Table 4

Carotis sinus syndrome

1. Cardiac inhibition	=	bradycardia
2. Vasodepression	=	fall in blood pressure

1st degree: no bradycardia, no hypotension

2nd degree: decrease of heart rate up to 20/min, asystole up to 2 s, a 10-20 mmHg fall in blood pressure

3rd degree: decrease of heart rate up to 30-50/min, asystole 2-3, fall in blood pressure of more than 30 mmHg

4th degree: asystole 3-5 s, fall in blood pressure of more than 50 mmHg

Remember:

Atropine test and carotid sinus massage may confirm a presumptive diagnosis. Without other evidence they do not lead to a final diagnosis. A somewhat longer pause following carotid sinus massage without adequate clinical signs does not give the indication for a pacemaker implantation.

Bradycardia due to a disorder of the SA node and atrium

Sinus bradycardia Sinus rhythm at a rate of less than 60/min with regular P waves preceeding the QRS complexes

Sinus arrhythmia Usually respiratory variation of sinus rate (accelerating with inspiration, slowing with expiration). Physiologic reaction in young people. In older people suggests dysfunction of the SA node. The respiratory arrhythmia is often absent in (diabetic) neuropathy of the heart

Sino-atrial block Regular discharges from the sinus node with failure in impulse propagation (exit block). Not all discharges from the sinus node lead to an atrial activation (Fig. 10)

Fig. 10

Sino-atrial block and its differential diagnosis

Differential diagnosis	**ECG (schematic)**
2nd degree SA block type 1 (Wenckebach)	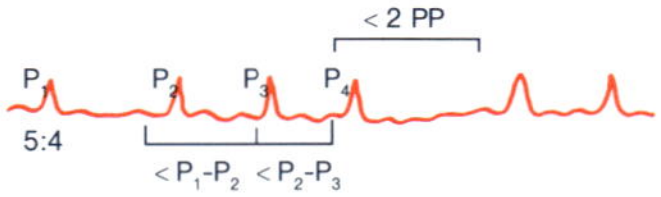
2nd degree SA block type 2, varying conduction ratio	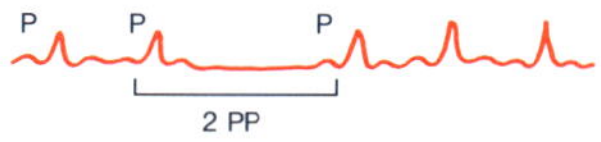
2nd degree SA block type 1, 3:2-(4:3) conduction ratio	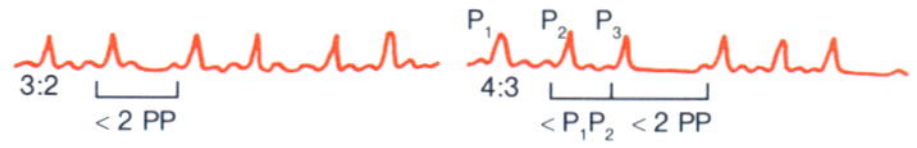
2nd degree SA block type 2, 3:2-(4:3) conduction ratio	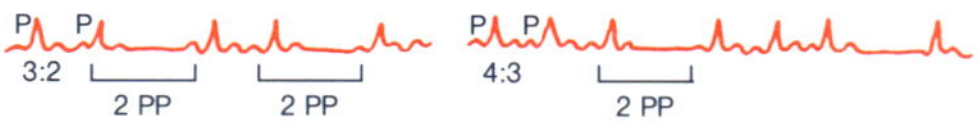
Sinus arrest	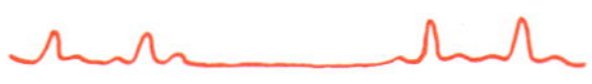
Sinus extrasystole	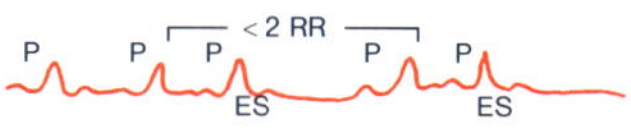
Blocked supraventricular extrasystole	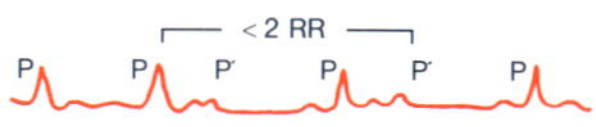

1st degree SA block: Not visible in the surface ECG

2nd degree SA block: Type Mobitz I (Wenckebach): Conduction from the SA node to the atrium is delayed, the time interval of delay increases from beat to beat. In the ECG: Progressive shortening of the PP interval until one complex drops out. The PR interval remains constant, the pause is shorter than a twofold PP distance

2nd degree SA block: Type Mobitz II: Sudden missing P waves and ventricular activation, the pause equals or exceeds the twofold PP distance. A constant conduction ratio of 2:1 or 3:1 appears as a sinus bradycardia. An intermittent 2:1 block appears with doubling of the PP intervals

3rd degree SA block: It has the appearance of a resting SA node (sinus arrest) with a pause of variable length and no relation to the inherent rhythm. The P waves and QRS complexes are absent until an escape rhythm supervenes

Sick sinus syndrome: See page 31

Bradycardia associated with disorders of the AV node

1st degree AV Block: Prolonged PR interval or AV conduction time to 0.2 s or more (Fig. 11)

Fig. 11

Schematic representation of AV block (modified by Haasis)

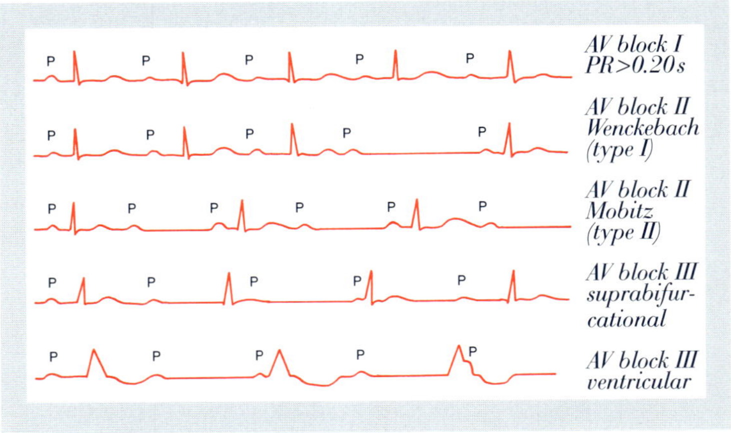

2nd degree AV block (type Mobitz I, Wenckebach): PR interval is somewhat lengthened. With each successive beat, the PR interval is lengthened and finally an impulse fails to reach the ventricles and a beat is dropped (absent QRS complex). The increase in the PR interval is most pronounced in the second cycle

2nd degree AV block type Mobitz II: Constant, usually normal AV conduction (PR interval) with repeated drop-out of the conduction in regular cycles (2:1, 3:1, 4:1)

3rd degree AV block (complete AV block, heart block): There is no relation between the regular activation of the atria and of the chambers. The atrial impulses cannot pass the AV node and fail to reach the ventricles. The atria and chambers beat totally independently. The atrial rhythm may be a normal sinus rhythm. Atrial tachycardias or atrial fibrillation may also be present

Proximal and distal block: The AV block is located either proximally (narrow QRS complexes) or distally (widened ventricular complexes). A more detailed differentiation can be obtained by recording the signal of the bundle of His (see p. 27, Table 5)

Table 5

Abnormal intraventricular conduction and recommendations regarding pacemaker therapy

	HV <55 ms	HV 60-89 ms	HV >90 ms
LBBB, RBBB AIVC	no	yes, if symptoms** are present	yes
RBBB + LAH LPH	no*	Yes, if symptoms** are present	yes
alternating LBBB/RBBB	rarely	yes	yes

* yes, if clear cardiac syncope
** after exclusion of extracardiac causes

Remark:

Though often published, this scheme still gives rise to criticism. The existence of typical clinical signs remains crucial before implantation of a pacemaker.

In order to distinguish between different HV intervals the invasive procedure of His bundle recording has to be performed. The HV interval is the period from the His deflection (H) and ventricular activation (V) (Fig. 13).

Abbreviations:

LBBB: Left bundle branch block
RBBB: Right bundle branch block
LAH : Left anterior fascicular hemiblock
LPH : Left posterior fascicular hemiblock
AIVC: Abnormal intra ventricular conduction

Stokes-Adams syndrome

Stokes-Adams attack:

Acute arrhythmias may lead to cerebral hypoperfusion and loss of consciousness. In brief reversible cases this is called syncope. In presence of bradycardia or ventricular arrhythmia with haemodynamic relevance irreversible lesions of the brain or heart may follow, even sudden death is possible. Causes of Stokes-Adams attacks are listed in Table 6

Table 6

Possible underlying arrhythmias in Stokes-Adams attacks

Tachycardias

Ventricular flutter or fibrillation

Rarely: Paroxysmal atrial fibrillation with high frequent tachyarrhythmia (mitral stenosis) and paroxysmal atrial flutter with regular conduction to the ventricles (uncommonly also 2:1 block)

Very rarely: Paroxysmal ventricular tachycardia and paroxysmal supraventricular tachycardia

Underlying diseases:
Myocardial ischaemia, myocarditis, in case of ventricular fibrillation or flutter among others digitalis, quinidine, procainamide, adrenalin (proarrhythmia)

Asystole

1. In sinus rhythm (often pre-existing partial SA or AV block):

   Inhibition of the impulse formation in the SA node (sinus arrest)

   Complete SA block
   Complete AV block
   } *termination by deblockage or development of a ventricular escape rhythm*

Reflex mechanism: Hypersensitive carotid sinus syndrome (cardiovagal, depressor, central type) blockade of the 3rd fascicle in pre-existing bifascicular block or block of the remaining bundle branch in right or left bundle branch block

2. In complete SA or AV block decrease of ventricular automatism or additonal disorders of impulse conduction

Underlying diseases:
Myocardial ischaemia, myocarditis, digitalis, primary degenerative disease of the specific myocardium

Severe bradycardia

e.g. sudden 2nd degree AV block (2:1 block or 4:1 block) and sinus bradycardia ("binodal" or "panconductional disease")

or sudden sinus bradycardia and pre-existing 2nd degree AV block

Heinecker 1980

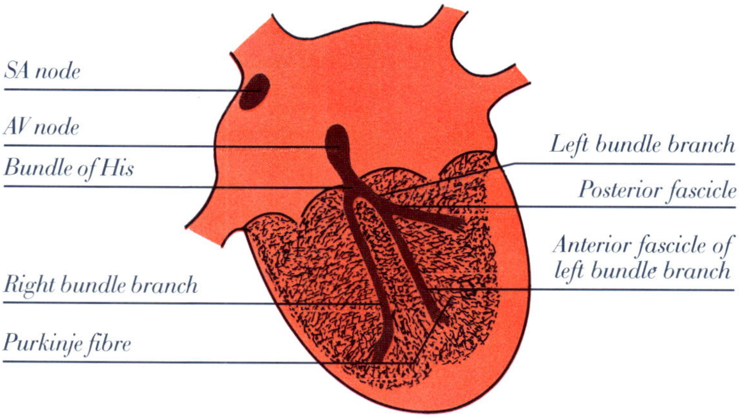

Fig. 12

The conduction system of the heart (by Sandøe)

Fig. 13

The His bundle electrogram (HBE) and intracardiac leads. Schematic drawing of the time intervals (modified from Sandøe)

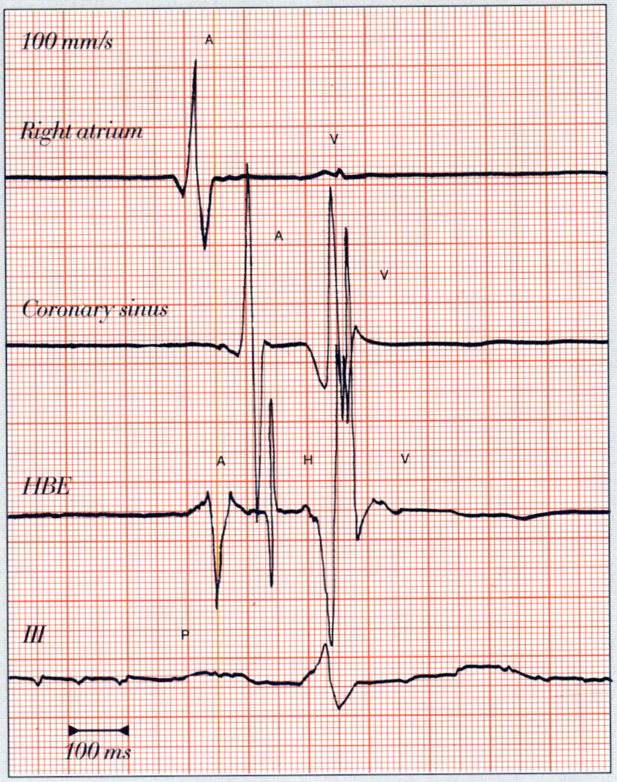

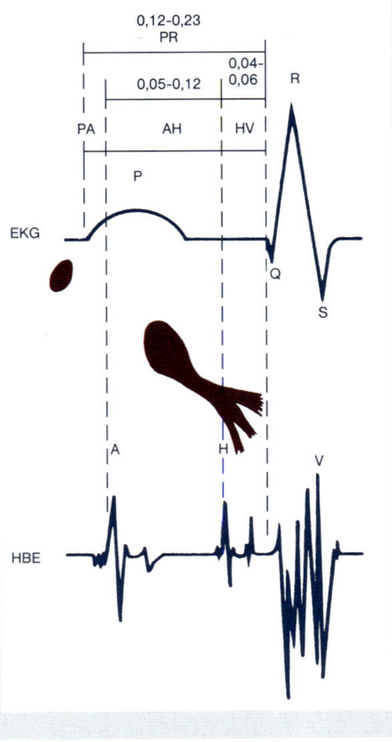

AV block

Recommendations regarding pacemaker therapy

	Localization intra-, infra-His	Localization AV node
1st degree AV block	yes, if symptoms	no
2nd degree AV block (type Mobitz)	yes	yes, if symptoms
3rd degree AV block	yes	yes, if symptoms

Table 7

Pacemaker therapy in different types of AV block. Clinical signs and symptoms have to be taken into consideration

The localization of the blockade in relation to the bundle of His can be determined only by an intracardiac electrogram and a His bundle recording. Mostly, a (complete) AV block and narrow QRS complex indicate a higher location, a widened QRS complex represents a lower site of blockade (infra-His) (see also Fig. 13).

Sick sinus syndrome

Synonym Bradycardia-tachycardia syndrome

Definition Alternation between periods of sinus nodal and junctional inertia and atrial or supraventricular tachyarrhythmias. Usually intermittent or permanent bradycardias may prevail and can be worsened by antiarrhythmic treatment for tachycardia

Type of arrhythmia In the sick sinus syndrome all types of supraventricular arrhythmias may occur: Supraventricular tachycardias, sinus bradycardias, sinus arrest, atrial fibrillation and flutter, often temporary and reversible

Diagnosis The diagnosis is based on Holter ECG, in some cases on electrophysiological testing. The indication for pacemaker therapy depends on the clinical situation, i.e. history, signs and symptoms

1 Disorder of the sinus node (sinus node dysfunction, sick sinus syndrome, bradycardia-tachycardia syndrome)

1.1 Indication

Intermittent or constant, marked sinus bradycardia related to the patients' complaints (symptomatic sinus bradycardia). Temporary and reversible manifestations of the sick sinus syndrome may be caused by drugs

1.2 Relative indication

Pronounced sinus bradycardia (spontaneous or due to drugs) at rates below 40/min with some evidence of a correlation between sinus bradycardia (or pause) and symptoms

1.3 No indication

Sinus bradycardias (or pauses) without complaints (asymptomatic sinus bradycardia), even if low rates are recorded

Pronounced sinus bradycardias or pauses during sleep (usually brief) with normal rate profile when awake

---

2 Carotid sinus syndrome (cardiodepressor type)

2.1 Indication

Recurrent (!) syncopes clearly related to an irritation of the carotid sinus (pressure on the neck, movements of the head to one side, looking up) which cause a short lasting asystole (SA node arrest, 3rd degree AV block).

2.2 Relative indication

Patients with recurrent otherwise unexplainable (!) syncopes, without clear relation to pressure on the carotid sinus but with abnormal response (more than 3s) to carotid sinus massage (so-called hypersensitive carotid sinus). Performing a carotid sinus massage the applied pressure should not suppress a palpable pulse of the ipsilateral temporal artery

2.3 No indication

Asymptomatic patients (hypersensitive carotid sinus)

Patients with atypical complaints and abnormal response to carotid sinus massage

Recurrent syncopes or almost complete syncopes if the vasodepressor type of hypersensitive carotid sinus predominates

---

3 Bradyarrhythmia in atrial fibrillation

3.1 Indication

Pronounced bradyarrhythmia with signs of cerebral underperfusion or significant intermittent relevant pauses of AV conduction (e.g. more than 3 s)

3.2 Relative indication

Bradyarrhythmia in heart failure

3.3. No indication

Pauses of the AV conduction of 2-3 s (asymptomatic or during sleep; common finding in the Holter ECG

---

4 Abnormal atrioventricular conduction

4.1 Indication

Acquired complete AV block (3rd degree), intermittent or permanent

Especially in the presence of symptoms or

with marked bradycardia (rate below 40/min) in patients free of symptoms or with an asystole of 3s or more or

in left and/or right heart failure or

with frequent ventricular ectopic beats or

with inadequate increase in rate on exercise testing with/without appearance of complex ventricular arrhythmias (see 2.2)

Intermittent or permanent 2nd degree AV block with clinical manifestation

2nd degree AV block type II (type Mobitz, generally distal blockade), permanent or intermittent without complaints

AV block following catheter ablation

4.2 Relative indication

3rd degree AV block without complaints, intermittent or permanent with escape rhythm of sufficient rate (more than 40/min)

2nd degree AV block type I (type Wenckebach) localized distal of the AV node (extremely rare, mainly supra-His), hardly asymptomatic

Transient 3rd degree AV block in catheter ablation (single observations suggest risk of permanent AV block in later life

4.3 No indication

1st degree AV block

2nd degree AV block (type Wenckebach) localized in the AV node, if asymptomatic

---

5 Congenital 3rd degree AV block

5.1 Indication

Slow escape rhythm (below 40-45/min) related to patients' symptoms. Inadequate rise in heart rate during exercise thus limiting the exercise capacity with/without appearance of ventricular arrhythmias on exercise (see 2)

5.2 Relative indication

Slow escape rhythm with symptoms at rest (lack of concentration, tiredness and weariness), but a sufficient rise in rate on exercise and adequate capacity for exertion

5.3 No indication

3rd degree AV block without complaints

---

6 Intraventricular blockade

Electrophysiological tests must be performed in uncertain situations

6.1 Indication

Bifascicular block with intermittent or permanent 2nd degree AV block (type Mobitz) or with intermittent 3rd degree AV block

6.2. Relative indication

Bi- or trifascicular block without a higher degree AV block causing syncopes (other causes of syncope are to be excluded)

Fascicular blockades with 1st degree AV block without complaints

6.3 No indication

Abnormal intraventricular conduction without evidence of a 2nd or 3rd degree AV block and without complaints (e.g., left anterior fascicular block with right bundle branch block)

---

7 Indication for permanent pacemaker implantation in the early postinfarction period (beginning about the 10th day)

Syncopes after infarction are often the result of ventricular tachycardias. Electrophysiological examination should be considered for further evaluation of the differential diagnosis

7.1 Indication

Patients with bradycardia below 50/min as a result of a persisting 2nd or 3rd degree AV block after infarction

7.2 Relative indication

Patients with a persistent 1st degree AV block und accompanying bundle branch block (which was not recorded before the infarction)

Patients with a temporary 2nd degree AV block and simultaneously a bundle branch block

7.3 No indication

Patients with transient abnormalities of the AV conduction during the period of acute infarction, without simultaneous abnormal ventricular conduction

Patients with a temporary AV block and simultaneously an isolated left anterior fascicular block

Patients with infarction related left anterior fascicular block without AV blockade

Selecting the pacing mode (modality)

In the following chapter an outline on the clinical impact of different pacing modes is attempted:

In general there are two modes available:

1. One-chamber devices (atrial or ventricular stimulation)
2. Dual-chamber devices (bifocal stimulation)

These devices work on demand at a constant, often programmable rate (AAI or VVI) or rate adapting (bifocal pacemaker with atrial sensing or rate adaption by special sensors, rate adapting stimulation in its proper sense)
Analogous to the valuation of the indication for pacemaker implantation, three categories are chosen for the selection of the pacing mode

Indication: Accepted form of stimulation

Relative indication: Controversial form of stimulation or borderline indication
No indication: Situations in which this form of stimulation should not be used

1 One-chamber devices

1.1 AAI (atrial stimulation, atrial sensing, inhibition)

1.1.1 Indication

Symptomatic disturbance of SA node function with intact AV conduction (normal PR interval, no 2nd or 3rd degree AV block in the Holter monitoring, Wenckebach point >140/min in atrial stimulation). Up to a quarter of the patients may have additional disturbances of atrioventricular or intraventricular conduction

1.1.2 Relative indication

Suppression of supraventricular (bradycardia/tachycardia syndrome) or ventricular arrhythmias

1.1.3 No indication

Pre-existing 1st or higher degree AV block and/or Wenckebach point below 140/min

Intermittent atrial fibrillation

1.2 VVI (ventricular stimulation, ventricular sensing, inhibition)

1.2.1 Indication

Any symptomatic bradyarrhythmia, especially when the atrial contractions are haemodynamically ineffective (atrial flutter or fibrillation) and/or there is no evidence of a pacemaker syndrome as a result of lost atrial contraction or a lack of atrioventricular synchronisation. The appearance of this syndrome cannot be completely excluded before implantation of a VVI pacemaker. The stimulation mode should be altered when the pulse generator is to be exchanged in patients with known pacemaker syndrome

1.2.2 Relative indication

Symptomatic bradycardias of any type with need for a simple pacing mode (e.g. with regard to age of patient)

1.2.3 No indication

Known pacemaker syndrome (in case of an exchange of the pulse generator) or similar symptoms in a foregoing temporary ventricular stimulation before the initial pacemaker implantation is planned

Indispensible contribution of the atrial contraction in heart failure

2 So-called physiological and rate adaptive ("biological") stimulation (bifocal and sensor controlled devices)

2.1 Indication

2.1.1 Exchange of pacemaker

In the presence of a pacemaker syndrome (change to bifocal stimulation)

In a reduced physical working capacity in daily life caused by an insufficient increase in rate: replacement of the non-rate adapting device (VVI or AAI) by a rate adapting one

In abnormal SA node function and intact AV conduction: Rate adapting VVI stimulation

In atrial fibrillation (bradyarrhythmia): Rate adapting VVI stimulation

In 3rd degree AV block and intact SA node function: Bifocal stimulation (DDD)

In case of an adequate increase in rate and reasonable physical working capacity: a non rate adapting device should be reimplanted

2.1.2 First implantation

3rd degree AV block with intact SA node function: Bifocal pacing (DDD)

3rd degree AV block with abnormal SA node function: Rate adapting VVI stimulation or rate adapting bifocal stimulation (DDD) (under current clinical investigation)

Bradyarrhythmia in atrial fibrillation with an inadequate increase in rate on moderate exercise associated with reduced physical working capacity (dyspnoea, weakness): Rate adapting VVI pacing

Symptomatic sinus bradycardia with an inadequate increase in rate producing symptoms on exercise:

With intact AV conduction: Rate adapting AAI stimulation

With abnormal AV conduction: Rate adapting stimulation either in VVI or DDD mode (when available)

Acquired iatrogenic 3rd degree block, e.g. following bundle of His ablation (rate adapting sensor controlled VVI stimulation)

2.1.3 No indication

Patients who are dependent on artificial pacing only intermittently (e.g. in carotid sinus syndrome or intermittent 3rd degree AV block)

Table 8

Nomenclature for pacemaker identification (For R (position 4) also: F)

Position	1	2	3	4	5
Category	site of pacing	site of sensing	response to sensing	programmability	anti-tachycardia function
Letter	A = atrium	0 = no sensing	0 = none	0 = none	B = burst
	V = ventricle	A = atrium	I = inhibited	P = programmable	S= scanning
	D=dual (A + V)	V = ventricle	T=triggered	(2 parameters at most	E= external control
	D=dual		D = dual	M = multiprogrammable	
			(I+T)	(R = rate adapting)	
				(C = communication)	
Example	V	V	I	M	
	D	D	D	M	
	A	A	I	M	B

Indications	• **Diagnosis of symptomatic arrhythmias**
Diagnosis of Arrhythmias	Bradycardia Tachycardia (supra- and ventricular origin) Evaluation of palpitations Transitory ischaemic attacks, Possibly after stroke
	• **Diagnosis of arrhythmias in suspected diseases** Coronary artery disease, especially after myocardial infarction After resuscitation Cardiomyopathies (hypertrophic and dilative type) Valvular heart disease, especially aortic stenosis Arterial hypertension Symptomatic mitral valve prolapse syndrome Pre-excitation syndrome, long QT syndrome
Symptoms	Evaluation of syncope, fainting and palpitations
Search for ischaemia	ST segment analysis for symptomatic ischaemia and asymptomatic (silent) ischaemia and for quantifying ischaemic events (Holter monitoring is not suitable for routine analysis of asymptomatic ischaemia)
Follow up	of medical treatment. Control of the efficiency of antiarrhythmic treatment, control of aggravation of arrhythmias by antiarrhythmic drugs (arrhythmogenic effect) **In detail:** Frequent and sustained complex ventricular arrhythmias, supra- and ventricular tachycardias. Atrial fibrillation, pre-excitation syndrome and abnormal conduction under antiarrhythmics
Follow up	of postoperative status (bypass surgery, PTCA, surgical treatment of arrhythmias)
Follow up	of pacemaker implantation (detection of pacemaker malfunction, detection of additional ventricular arrhythmias)

Conditions for ambulatory monitoring analysis

Recording over at least 24 hours

Recording of at least 2 monitoring leads

Correct lead position

Availability of a continuous print out of the ECG

Limits for frequency between 0.05/s and 100/s if possible

Sufficient linearity and baseline stability

Visual control of the ECG by 1:1 reprints

Electrode placement

Location of electrodes (Fig. 14, 15)

Removal of hair, fat and the most superfi cial layer of the skin

Fixation of the electrodes and wires

Check of postural and motional constancy

Calibration

Start

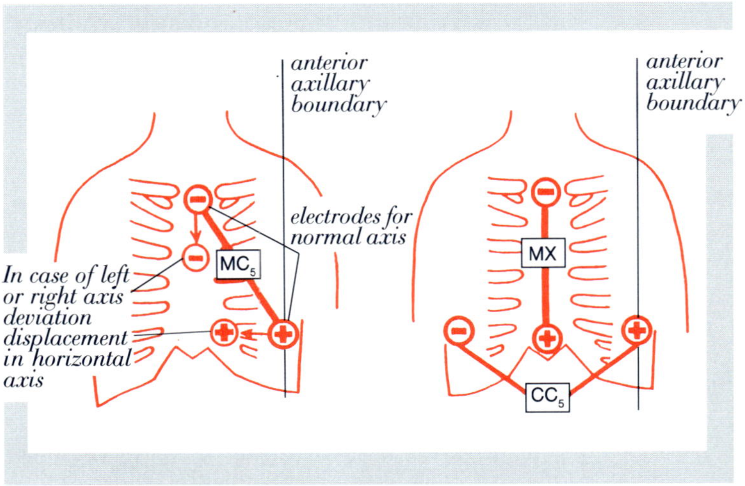

On the left side a right and left precordial lead. (V_2 and V_5): Different electrode over the 5th intercostal space at the anterior axillary boundary, the indifferent electrode over the manubrium sterni.

In horizontal axis: displacement of the indifferent electrode caudally.
In vertical axis: displacement of the different electrode medially.

On the right side another variation with the indifferent electrode over the manubrium sterni (M) and the different electrode over the xiphoid processus (X), the second variation follows the CC5 scheme.

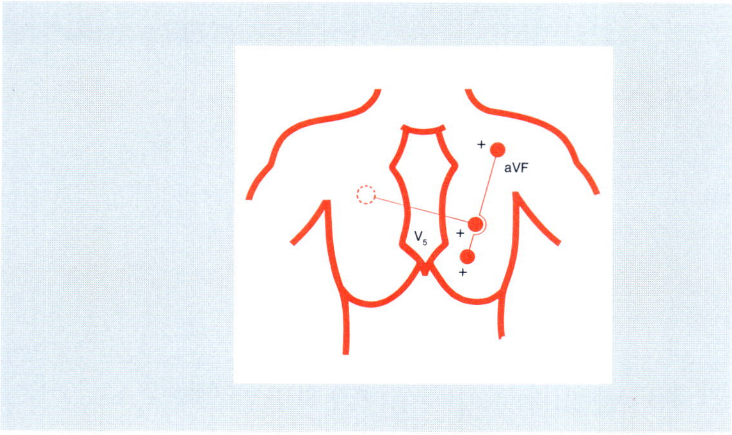

Fig. 15

Scheme of leads for analysis of the ST segment with modified aVF/V_5 scheme (modified by v. Olshausen and Höpp).

Causes of possible artifacts

- Muscular artifacts, detachment of electrodes
- Movement artifacts, zero drift
- Defect in tape transport
- Incomplete erasing of the tape

Conditions for evaluation

- Adequate training of the performing staff
- Adequate technical equipment
- Observance of quality control
- Documentation

Classification according to frequency

PACs	
Rare	<15/hour
Occasional	15 to 29/hour
Frequent	>30/hour
SVTs	
Rare	<1 episode every 6 months
Occasional	>1 episode every 3 to 6 months
Frequent	>1 episode/month
Daily	daily recurrences of SVT
Incessant	Frequent, daily, recurrence of SVT with rare periods of sinus rhythm intervening (SVT >10 % a day)
Non-sustained	At least 3 consecutive PACs at a rate >100 beats/min but selfterminating in <2 minutes
Sustained	SVT lasting >2 minutes or requiring termination before that time due to haemodynamic compromise

PACs = premature atrial contractions
SVT = supraventricular tachycardia

(Naccarelli, 1986)

Classification of supraventricular arrhythmias

1. Sinus arrhythmias
2. Atrial arrhythmias
3. AV node or junctional arrhythmias

- Sinus arrhythmia
  Sinus rhythm with cyclic undulation of the rate with respiration (physiological): Increase in rate with inspiration and decrease in rate with expiration

- Supraventricular or atrial extrasystoles
  Premature P wave with subsequent QRS complex. The QRS complex is not widened or bizarre. There is a fixed relation to the preceding discharge, the subsequent pause is not compensatory (Fig. 16)

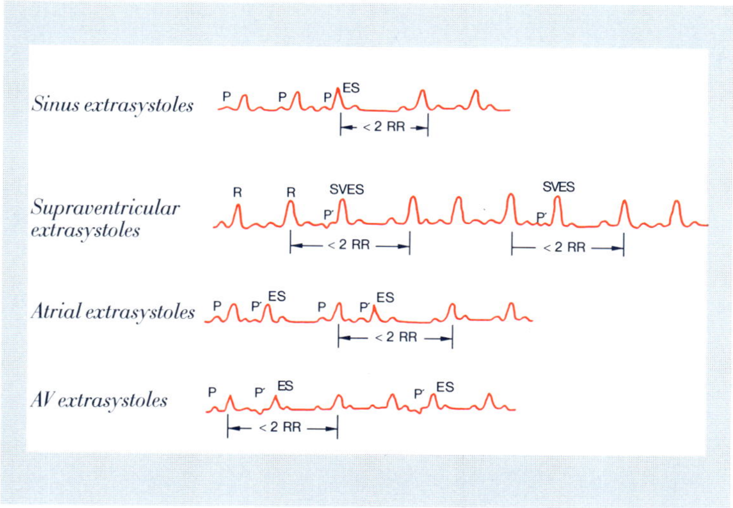

Fig. 16

Supraventricular extrasystoles

- Atrial arrhythmias:

  Atrial extrasystoles: Premature P wave (the PP interval shorter than the normal one) with subsequent normal QRST complex. The length of the following pause is different to a normal PP distance

  Upper atrial origin: The vector of the P wave is normal, positive P in I and aVF

  Lower atrial origin: The P wave is negative in II, III, aVF. The PR interval is shorter than that of a sinus beat. These extrasystoles are difficult, almost impossible to distinguish from junctional extra beats

  Blocked atrial extrasystoles: A premature P wave shortly after a QRS complex. There is no conduction to the ventricle because of the AV node which is still refractory

  Wandering pacemaker: Change from regular to irregular ventricular rhythms. Each QRS complex is preceded by a P wave of varying contour and PR interval

- Atrial tachycardia:
  Regular atrial activation, constant PP interval with an atrial rate of about 160-220/min. The P wave originates from upper or lower regions of the atrium (see above)

  Atrial tachycardia with 1:1 conduction ratio: Each P wave is followed by a QRS complex. Formally sometimes difficult to distinguish from sinus tachycardia. Diagnosis often established by further ECG recordings or by oesophageal or intracardiac ECG

  Atrial tachycardia with block: Atrial tachycardia with varying conduction ratio and inconstant relationship between P waves and QRS complexes

- Atrial flutter:
  Regular P waves (rate 260-320/min) mostly "sawtooth appearance" of the P waves in II, III, V_1, aVF, usually 2:1 or 3-4:1 conduction. By vagal manoeuvers "unmasking" into 2:1 conduction due to a higher degree of blockade making the atrial flutter easier to recognize. Atrial flutter with 2:1 conduction ratio is often mistaken for sinus tachycardia

- Atrial fibrillation:
  No regular P waves, rather an uneven zero line, varying distances of the QRS complexes

- AV junctional rhythms:
  Junctional ectopic discharges: Formally identical to supraventricular extrasystoles from the lower atrium

  Junctional rhythm: Regular atrial rhythm with 1:1 conduction at a rate of 50-100/min. Negative P waves in II, III, aVF. The PR interval is short, rarely normal and sometimes can be seen after the QRS complex

  Junctional tachycardia: Identical with junctional rhythm but at a rate of 120-200/min

Remember: Atrial tachycardia and junctional tachycardia are the usual paroxysmal tachycardias. Their appearance is intermittent at a rate of about 170-220/min. Often vagal manoeuvres can interrupt these supraventricular tachycardias.

- Differential diagnosis of supraventricular arrhythmias or narrow - QRS tachycardia (Fig. 17):
  Sinus, atrial or AV extrasystoles
  Blocked atrial extrasystoles
  Alternation of sinus rhythm and AV rhythm (dissociation)
  Supraventricular, atrial or AV parasystole
  Altering site of automaticity
  AV escape rhythm, junctional escape rhythm

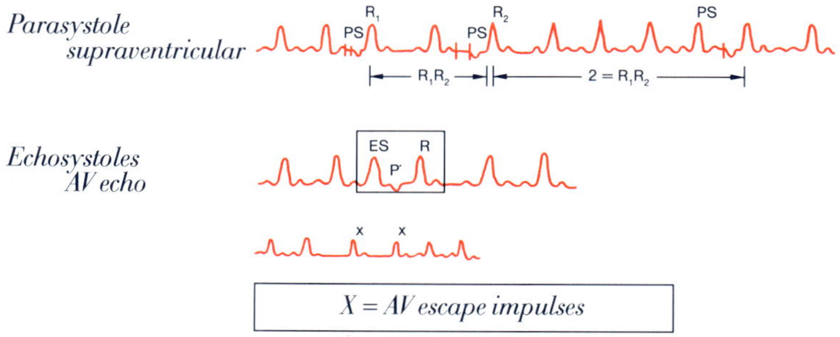

Fig. 17

Differential diagnosis supraventricular arrythmias

Definition of parasystole

There are non-fixed coupling intervals between normal and extra beats. In between the parasystolic beats there are simple multiples of the same integer. Fusion complexes occur (normal and parasystolic activation meet).

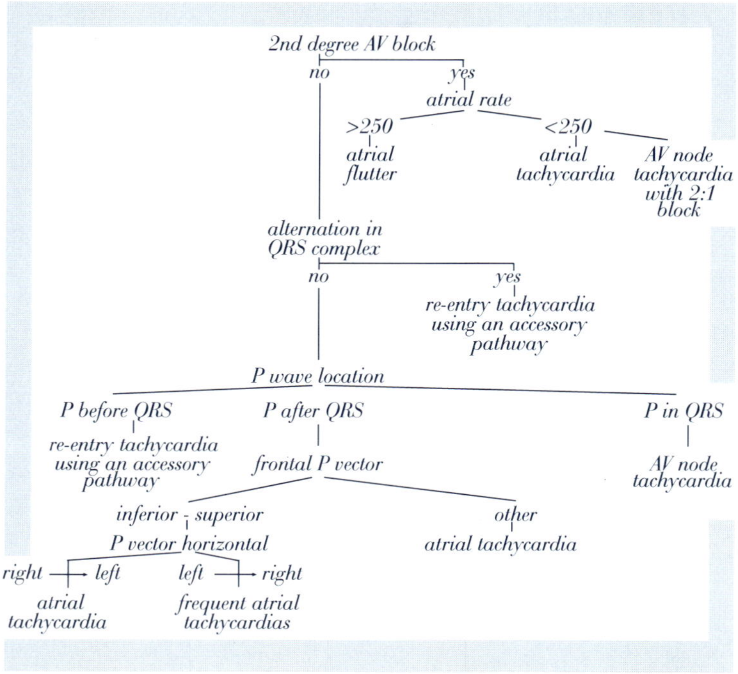

Fig. 18

Tachycardia with narrow QRS complex: electrocardiographic differential diagnosis

Causes

Arrhythmias are based on an arrhythmogenic substrate, on triggering factors and modulating factors (Fig. 19). The different mechanisms of impulse formation are shown in Table 9.

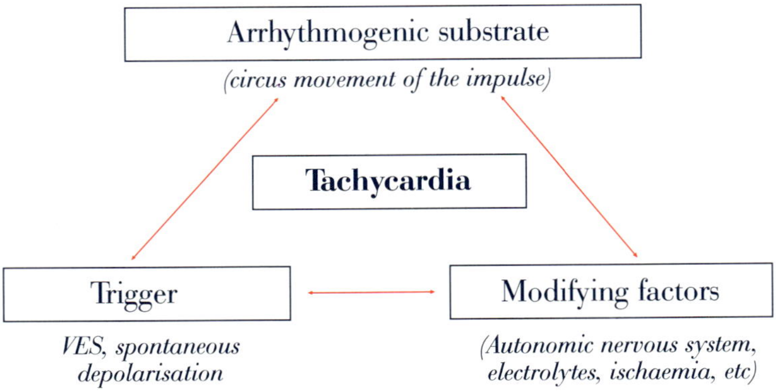

Fig. 19

Pathophysiological factors in formation of arrhythmias (modified by Brugada)

Table 9

Formation of arrhythmias

I. Abnormal impulse formation
   Abnormal automaticity
   Triggered activity
   Early or delayed afterdepolarisation

II. Abnormal impulse conduction
   Delay and block (SA, AV)
   Unidirectional block and re-entry
   Reentry: Random or regular summation and inhibition
   Conduction block (electrotonic transmission and reflection)

III. Simultaneous abnormality of impulse formation and propagation
   Parasystole
   Slow conduction because of phase 4 depolarisation

Classification Ventricular arrhythmias can be divided up as follows:

Ventricular extrasystoles of various appearances

Parasystole

Idioventricular rhythm

Ventricular tachycardia, ventricular flutter and fibrillation.

Definitions Ventricular extrasystole (VES)

A premature ventricular complex with fixed coupling to the preceding activation of the same chamber. The premature beat is commonly followed by a postextrasystolic pause (compensatory pause), thus the interval between two normal beats equals two RR intervals. Exceptions are interpolated extrasystoles.

Characteristics of extrasystoles

Prematurity

Fixed coupling interval

Bizarre shape of the QRS complex

Secondary T and ST alterations

Distinct sequence of conduction and pattern of distribution

Effect on the basic rhythm

AV dissociation possible

Retrograde conduction possible

Differentiation

Supraventricular extrasystole with aberrance

Atrial fibrillation with intermittent aberrance

Intermittent pre-excitation (seldom)

Parasystole, occasionally alternating with extrasystoles

Rate dependent left bundle branch block

Bigeminy Normal beats and extrasystoles are alternating

Trigeminy Each normal beat is followed by two extrasystoles. One extrasystole after two or three normal beats is called 2:1 and 3:1 extrasystole respectively

Forms Unifocal: Extrasystoles of the same configuration

Multifocal: Extrasystoles different in form or main vector (direction of deflection).

Terms like monomorphic/polymorphic or monotopic/polytopic are also in use and suggest different sites of origin in the myocardium.

Parasystole Extra beats with nonfixed coupling interval. There is a mathematical relationship between ectopic beats. Fusion complexes occur

Frequent extrasystoles Frequent extrasystoles are defined as 10 or more extrasystoles per hour

---

Repetitive extrasystoles or repetitive ventricular responses:

Two or more consecutive ventricular extrasystoles up to ventricular tachycardia

Couplet Two consecutive extrasystoles

Remember:

Couplet is: Two successive lines of verse, equal in length and with rhyme. Probably couplet means "coupling" of two extrasystoles. The term is enduring despite its linguistic inaccuracy. Synonym: Pair

Run Three to five consecutive extrasystoles

Ventricular tachycardia Sustained or non-sustained ventricular tachycardia:

Six or more consecutive ventricular extrasystoles lasting less than 30 seconds with spontaneous termination. As a rule no haemodynamic impairment is present. The rate above 100/min and the width of the QRS complex more than 120 ms

Sustained ventricular tachycardia:

Ventricular tachycardia lasting more than 30 s, requiring termination by medical or electrical treatment (intervention). Haemodynamic compromise is present

Remember:

Ventricular tachycardias are often met with fusion complexes or escape beats. These ventricular complexes are formally an intermediate type of normal beats and extrasystoles

Atypical ventricular tachycardia (Torsade de pointes): Ventricular tachycardia with continuous undulation or spindle-shaped groupings of the QRS complexes around the isoelectric line

Ventricular flutter Homogeneous, regular consecutive ventricular complexes with widenend and usually deformed QRS complexes at a rate of 180-250/min. Spontaneous termination is possible, but deterioration to ventricular fibrillation is frequent

Ventricular fibrillation Electrical activation of the myocardium in a rapid sequence, with irregular form and amplitude, no main direction of the deflections, rate around 250-400/min, functionally identical to cardiac arrest

---

Special forms of extrasystoles

Escape rhythm Escape rhythm appears when the normal sinus impulse does not arrive at the AV node or ventricle and a regular rhythm is originated by the AV node or the ventricle (junctional rhythm, idioventricular rhythm)

Possible causes: Primary failure of the SA node (arrest, sinus bradycardia), conduction disturbances in the atrium or AV node (SA or AV block). Thus the escape rhythm is a type of rescuing beat

Concealed ventricular bigeminy or trigemy Beside the basic rhythm a bigeminy (trigeminy) exists that cannot be detected in the surface ECG but results in a disturbed conduction in the subsequent beat. This is due to a changing exit block which allows impulse formation only at distinct intervals. These are typical intervals between normal beats and extrasystoles with an even number of sinus beats in between the extrasystoles (bigeminy) or they follow the rule 3n + 2, i.e. three sinus beats or a multiply plus two beats (trigeminy; VES each time after 2, 5, 8, 11, 14...beats)

Intermittent ventricular parasystole The same criteria as above apply for intermittent ventricular parasystole. Fusion-complexes are more frequent

Rule of bigeminy Tendency of premature ventricular beats to follow a long preceding RR interval. The following postextrasystolic pause causes another long RR interval, this favours the development of another extrasystole resulting in bigeminy

Aberration (Intermittent) aberrant ventricular conduction is the abnormal spread of an impulse originating in the atria or AV junction through an abnormal ventricular conduction pathway, which is partly in a refractory state. The ventricular complexes are bizarre and may also appear in a bundle branch block configuration

Ashman's phenomenon Aberration during ventricular conduction with a short cycle following a long RR interval. Aberration frequently occurs in atrial fibrillation (Fig. 20)

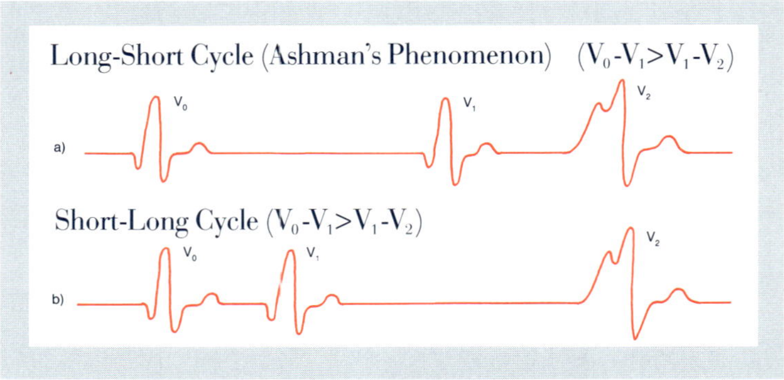

Fig. 20

Schematic representation:
a) Long-short cycle sequence with V_0-V_1 greater than V_1-V_2 (Ashman's phenomenon) suggesting aberration.
b) Short-long cycle sequence with V_0-V_1 less than V_1-V_2, suggesting ventricular extrasystole

Rate dependent left bundle branch block In some cases there is, at an increased rate of the basic rhythm, a widened and deformed ventricular complex with a bundle branch block pattern. The diagnosis of rate-dependent bundle branch block is easy with sinus rhythm. In atrial fibrillation this has to be differentiated from tachycardia with widened ventricular complex. The typical feature of a rate dependent bundle branch block is its appearance or disappearance above or below a certain rate, for example around 100-120/min

Efficacy control of treatment by ambulatory monitoring

Supraventricular arrhythmias	Infrequent supraventricular arrhythmias: Less than 15 min/day, 30% decrease in heart rate or time in supraventricular tachycardias Frequent supraventricular arrhythmias: Reduction to less than 20% = notable symptomatic improvement
Ventricular arrhythmias	80% reduction of ventricular extrasystoles (65-85%) 90% reduction of pairs/couplets/runs (75-90) Complete suppression of ventricular tachycardias (90-100%)
Proarrhythmic effect	(Arrhythmogenic effect or aggravation) Table 10

Table 10

Terminology for Proarrhythmia (modified from Horowitz, 1987)

Arrhythmogenesis:
Creation of arrhytmia by any cause

Proarrhythmia:
Drug-induced (primarily by antiarrhythmic drugs) arrhythmogenesis

Provocation of arrhythmia:
Creation by drugs of a new arrhythmia

Aggravation of arrhythmia:
Worsening by drugs of previously documented arrhythmia

Types of proarrhythmia:
Bradycardias (SA, AV node): e.g. digitalis, beta-blocker, calcium antagonists, antiarrhythmic drugs
Tachycardias: Supraventricular, ventricular

Criteria of proarrhythmia:

Torsade de pointes with QT prolongation

New onset of sustained, uniform ventricular tachycardia (conversion of nonsustained ventricular tachycardia to sustained ventricular tachycardia)

New, multiform, sustained ventricular tachycardia without QT prolongation

Increased frequency of ventricular premature complexes or repetitive forms

Responses to programmed electrical stimulation:

Conversion of non-sustained to sustained ventricular tachycardia

Increased rate of ventricular tachycardia

Initiation of ventricular tachycardia with fewer premature stimuli

Criteria of proarrhythmia (cont.):

4-fold increase in ventricular extrasystole

10-fold increase in repetitive forms

Conversion of nonsustained ventricular tachycardia to sustained ventricular tachycardia

New onset of ventricular tachycardias, flutter or fibrillation.

Atypical ventricular tachycardia (torsade de pointes)

Aggravation is not uncommon with prolongation of the QT interval by antiarrhythmic drugs. The QT interval not corrected for rate should not exceed 500 to 550 ms, or 450 ms or 120% for the corrected QT.

Calculation of the QT duration (corrected for rate, QTc) with the Bazett's formula:

$$QTc = \frac{QT}{\sqrt{\text{RR interval}}}$$ (normal value: Less than 0.44 s)

Recommendations for antiarrhythmic treatment

During treatment with antiarrhythmic drugs the QT interval should not exceed 120%, the QRS width should not increase more than 25%.

Recommendations for avoidance of arrhythmias caused by QT prolongation with quinidine-like antiarrhythmic drugs (mandatory in antiarrhythmic therapy):

Checking of the ECG 1 hour after the first dose.

Checking of the ECG within the first week after initiation of therapy.

Discontinuation of treatment if QT interval exceeds 120%

Ventricular arrhythmia and prognosis

According to current standards the prognosis of patients with ventricular arrhythmias is worsened with

- organic heart disease
- impaired left ventricular function (ejection fraction less than 35%)
- high incidence of ventricular extrasystoles (>10/h) and with complex ventricular arrhythmias
- documented syncopes or resuscitation prior to therapy

Classification of ventricular arrhythmias

Various criteria have been proposed for the classification of ventricular arrhythmia. The classification by Lown has found wide propagation. Using Lown's classification the total number of extrasystoles per hour has to be counted. With regard to clinical relevance more than 10 extrasystoles/hour means a worsened prognosis

Lown Classification : Table 11, 12

Table 11

Classification of ventricular extrasystoles

0	No ventricular extrasystoles (VES)
Ia	Occasional ventricular extrasystoles (<1/min, <30/hour)
Ib	Occasional ventricular estrasystoles (>1/min, <30/min)
II	Frequent ventricular extrasystoles (>30/min)
III	Multiform ventricular extrasystoles
IV	Repetitive ventricular extrasystoles
IVa	Pairs (couplets) of ventricular extrasystoles
IVb	Runs of three or more consecutive extrasystoles
V	Early falling in of ventricular extrasystoles (prematurity index* below 1)

* [Calculation of the prematurity index = $\frac{Q_N Q_{VES}}{QT_N}$

$Q_N Q_{VES}$ = interval from Q_N (Q of the normal beat prior to the VES) until QVES (Q of the extrasystole)

QT_N = QT interval (onset Q to end of T) of the normal beat]

Table 12

Example of the analysis of a Holter ECG

Holter ECG record	
0^3	No arrhythmia during 3 hours
$1A^0$	No arrhythmia type 1A
$1B^4$	Occasional VES (>1/hour) during 4 hours
2^6_{760}	Grade 2 during 6 hours, in total 760
3^6_2	Grade 3 during 6 hours, 2 forms
$4A^2_3$	Grade 4 during 2 hours (highest incidence in 1 hour: 3)
$4B^2_{4-7}$	During 2 hours 4 times, longest duration: 7 cycles
5^1_3	During 1 hour 3 times

Scheme showing the classification of ventricular extrasystoles according to LOWN with some examples (modified from Bethge). This classification should be interpreted with additional recordings of the total number of extrasystoles.

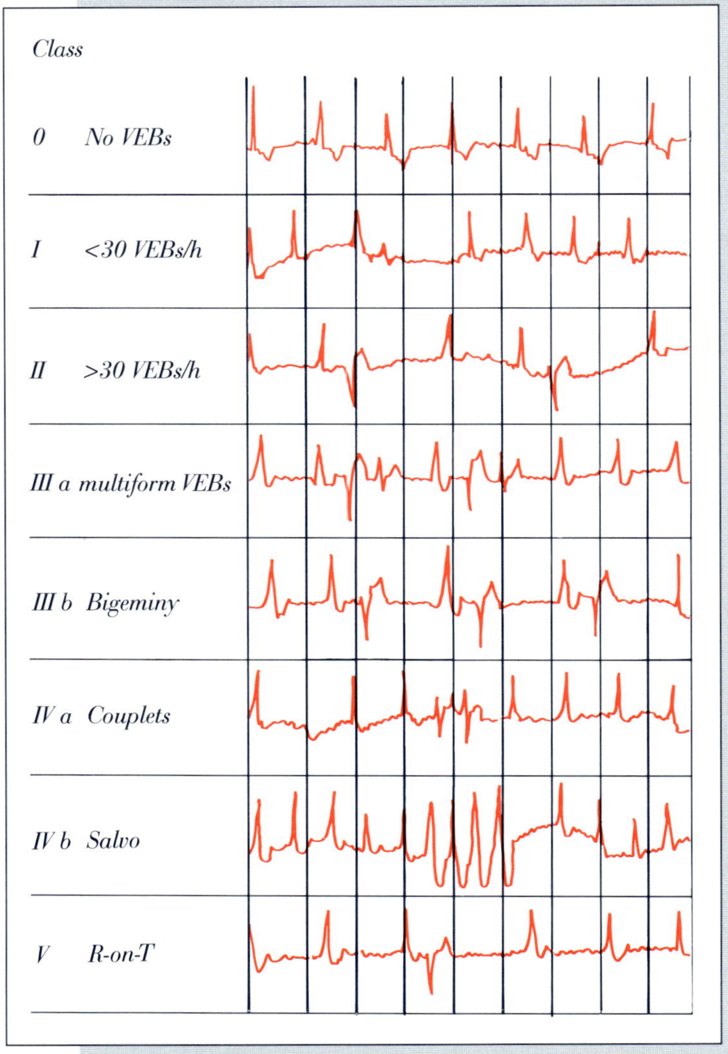

Table 13

Classification by Myerburg wihout a hierarchic subdivision

	Frequency		Form
0	none	A:	uniform or unifocal
I	very occasional (<1/hour)	B:	multiform or multifocal
II	occasional (1-9/hour)	C:	repetitive form
III	increased (10-29/hour)	D:	nonsustained ventricular tachycardia
IV	frequent (>30/hour)	E:	sustained ventricular tachycardia

According to recent investigations and consensus conferences with respect to the results of the CAST study there is a tendency towards classifications with more clinical impact (Table 14, 15).

Table 14

Clinical classification of ventricular arrhythmias

	Benign	Potentially hazardous	Malign
Sudden death risk	Minimal	Moderate	High
Symptoms	Palpitations on routine check	Palpitations on routine check	Palpitations Syncope Cardiac arrest
Cardiac disease	Most absent	Present	Present
Haemodynamic effect	Low	Moderate	High
Myocardial scars and/or hypertrophy	Absent	Present	Present
Incidence of VES	Low	Moderate	High
Repetitive VES	Absent	Frequent Nonsustained	Frequent Sustained
Therapeutic aim	Relief of symptoms	Symptomatic Reduction of arrhythmia Prevent sudden death	Relief of symptoms Reduction of arrhythmia Prevent sudden death

Bigger, 1984

Table 15

Non-hierarchic classification of ventricular arrhythmias

Ventricular extrasystoles (rare, frequent, complex, asymptomatic ventricular tachycardia)	**Sustained symptomatic ventricular tachycardia**	**Ventricular fibrillation**
Increase with age and with severity of heart disease. No independent marker of prognostic value but indicator of heart disease	As a rule indicator of severe heart disease, no sequelae of preceding "complex" arrhythmias	As a rule an electrical event without clear relation to preceding ventricular arrhythmias, may result from a sustained ventricular tachycardia

Surawicz, 1989

Table 16

Possible causes of arrhythmogenic cardiac disorders

Name of disorder	**Pathophysiology**	**Type of arrhythmia**
Pre-excitation syndrome	Accesory AV conduction pathway	Supraventricular tachycardia
Lenègre's and Lev's diseases	Fibrotic changes in the AV conduction and the intraventricular conduction system	AV block bundle branch block
Sick sinus syndrome	Fibrosis in the atrial wall and in the SA node area	Tachycardia or bradycardia
Long QT syndrome	Congenital, drug-induced metabolic changes and others	Ventricular tachycardia torsade de pointes
Arrhythmogenic right ventricular dysplasia	Adipose and fibrous infiltrations of the myocardial wall of the right ventricle	Ventricular tachycardia often with a left bundle branch block pattern
Antiarrhythmic treatment	Abnormal repolarisation	Ventricular tachycardia increased ventricular extrasystoles

Tachycardia with wide QRS-complex:

Differential diagnosis of aberrant ventricular conduction versus ventricular origin of tachycardia.

Definition: Aberrant ventricular conduction (or aberrancy) is the temporary, abnormal intraventricular conduction or supraventricular impulses, usually due to a change in cycle length (Marriot, 1988).

Aberrancy often occurs as a temporary phenomenon during an otherwise regular rhythm or during atrial fibrillation.

Mechanism: Aberration depends on an unequal refractoriness of the intraventricular conduction system. An early or premature supraventricular impulse finds parts of the bundle branches responsive and parts refractory. Conduction occurs resulting in a right bundle branch pattern in most cases (80 %). A hemiblock may complicate this bundle branch configuration. Left bundle branch pattern occurs less often (about 20 %).

Diagnosis: Differentiation is shown in Table 17. In general, tachycardia with wide QRS-complex should be interpreted as ventricular origin unless there are typical signs of another origin. Differentiation depends on form, duration and axis deviation of the QRS complex and of the R-wave in the frontal plane. Further help is presented by capture or fusion beats (indicationg ventricular origin).

Diagnosis is improved and more reliable via the esophagus lead or the intracardiac ECG.

Therapy:	Treatment depends on the actual hemodynamic situation and the underlying cardiac disease. In some cases, electrical therapy may be necessary (cardioversion, overstimulation). Drug therapy can be initiated if there is no compromized circulatory situation. The drugs preferred in this situation are those, which are effective in the preexcitation syndrome, e.g. propafenon, ajmaline (available only in Europe) and others, as well as type III antiarrhythmics.

Table 17

Differentiation of aberrant ventricular conduction versus ventricular origin in tachycardia with wide QRS-complex.

Supraventricular origin (Aberrancy)	Regular relation between P and QRS and between QRS and P, Right bundle branch pattern, QRS more narrow than 0.13ms, regular distances between QRS complexes, in case of atrial fibrillation no compensatory pause. Initial vector identical with that of flanking conducted beats.
Ventricular origin:	VA-dissociation, intermittent atrio-ventricular conduction, (capture beats, fusion beats), fixed coupling, shorter preceding cycle ("short-long-cycle"), especially in atrial fibrillation.

Special remarks	Aberration	Ventricular origin
RBBB V_1 V_6	Triphasic contour (rsR' or rSr', RSR') S<R	mono- or biphasic contour notched configuration (qR) S >R
LBBB R in V_1 S in V_{2-6} R axis	R in V_1 narrow or not present less deep than in V_1 normal, only minimal right axis deviation	wide ≥ 0.16 deeper than in V_1 right axis deviation −90° to −180°
QRS-duration	0.12s, <0.14s	>0.14s
Main vector in frontal plane	discordant from V_1 to V_6	Concordant from V_1 to V_6

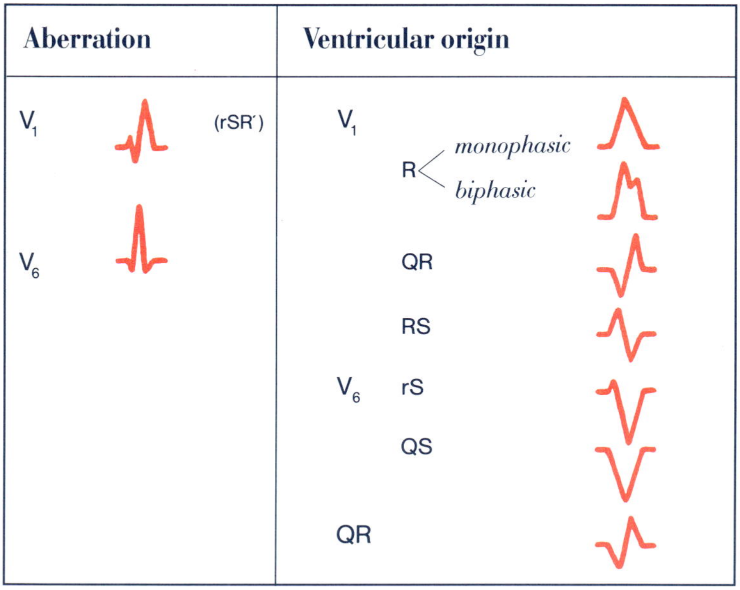

Fig. 21

Schematic presentation of tachycardia with wide QRS-complex

Indications for ergometry

Diagnostic indication:

Evaluation of functional physical capacity of patients, healthy subjects, or athletes

Evaluation of physical fitness for special tasks or special occupations (e.g., pilots, firemen, lorry drivers, divers)

Investigations of physical fitness (research only)

Screening for suspected latent diseases (clinical indication):

Noninvasive

Coronary artery disease, hypertension, hyperkinetic circulation, exercise-induced asthma

Invasive

Left ventricular failure, latent pulmonary hypertension, disturbed respiratory gas exchange

Recommendation for exercise testing:

In daily life

Sports activities (e.g. coronary rehabilitation),
before starting physical training in patients with cardiac and pulmonary diseases and with hypertension

Control of therapy

Contraindications of ergometry

Prognostic evaluation

Diseases of the heart and circulation with pronounced compromised cardiopulmonary function (severe heart failure in valvular disease, cardiomyopathy, coronary artery disease), severe arrhythmias, thrombosis, uncontrolled hypertension, severe pulmonary hypertension, symptomatic aortic stenosis, resting blood pressure >180 mmHg. Severe diseases of other organs (such as pneumonia, cholecystitis, acute hepatitis, acute nephritis)

Ergometry under clinical conditions:

Congenital or acquired valvular disease. Valvular disease with syncopes, early postinfarct period (10-20 days). Uncontrolled hypertension. 2nd to 3rd degree AV block, left bundle branch block

Complex arrhythmias at a former ergometry. Unstable angina pectoris

The early period after angioplasty or bypass surgery of the coronary arteries

Table 17

Recommendation for a programme for exercise testing (bicycle testing)

Field of application	Initial workload (W)	Increment
GP office, clinic, 'routine ergometry' occupational medicine	50 75-100 (good fitness)	25 W per 2 min
GP office, clinic, nuclear cardiology	50 (reduced fitness: 25 W)	25 W per 2 min expert opinion,
Pnęumology (in case of right heart catheterisation and blood gas analysis)	(25) 50	25 W per 5 min
Pediatric stress testing	1 W per kg* for 3 min	0.5 W per kg*
Sports medicine	50 (female) 100 (male) or 150	50 W per 3 min 25 W in the range of exhaustion

Preparatory conditions: Pretest period of 5 min. Resting values are obtained within the 3 preceding minutes before the test. Recovery period: 6 minutes. Recordings of blood pressure, heart rate and ECG. (= body weight)*

Test programme

Initial workload:	25, 50 W (or 100, 150 W)
Exercise steps:	25W per 2 min (or 50W)
Pretest and recovery period:	6 min each, at least 3 test stages
Total duration:	Less than 15 min
Pedal rate:	60-70/min (submax.) 60-100/min (max.)

Conditions for performing exercise testing

Examination and tests:

History, clinical examination, resting exercise testing ECG, resting blood pressure, drug history.

Methodology:

Room temperature (18-24°C), relative humidity (30-60%), deviations from these conditions must be recorded.

Calibration of the ergometer! Continuous recording of the ECG throughout the test or monitoring of ECG, pedal rate in the recommended range (60-70/min; 60-90/min for maximal workload), monitoring of blood pressure during exercise testing

Subjects:
Body temperature within the normal range. No food intake and no strenuous physical effort in the last 2 hours before ergometry

No alcohol or nicotine within the last 12 hours before testing

Drugs:
Sufficiently long pause (e.g., beta-blockers, digitalis)

Staff:
Presence of an experienced physician (certified qualification)

Signs of pathological alteration in the exercise ECG

The pathological ECG during exercise

ST segment depression (ischaemic alterations in response)

ST segment depression: Horizontal or downsloping 0.06 to 0.08 s after J point >0.1mV; J point depression >0.1 mV and ST depression >0.1 mV in 0.06 and 0.08 s after J points

J point depression and slowly upsloping ST segment >0.2 mV 0.06 to 0.08s after J

J point depression

Depression more than 0.2 mV probably abnormal response

ST segment elevation

Abnormal response: >0.1 mV

Significance:

Without previous infarction: Proximal stenosis of left anterior descending artery, coronary spasm (Prinzmetal angina)

With previous infarction: Sign of regional wall motion abnormality (a-, hypo-, dyskinesia, aneurysm)

Rhythm and conduction disturbances in the exercise ECG

- Supraventricular premature beats >5/min, multifocal appearance, intermittent or new, exercise-induced atrial fibrillation or flutter, paroxysmal atrial tachycardia
- Complex ventricular arrhythmias, idioventricular rhythm, ventricular runs or tachycardias
- Abnormalities of impulse formation and conduction. New 2nd and 3rd degree SA block, new 2nd and 3rd degree AV block
- Right bundle branch block, monofascicular block, bifascicular block, left bundle branch block (all new, also rate-dependent block)

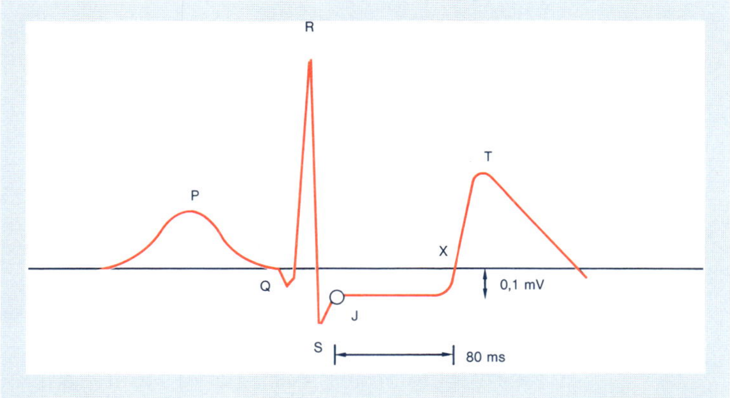

Fig. 22

Determination of segments and points in the exercise ECG

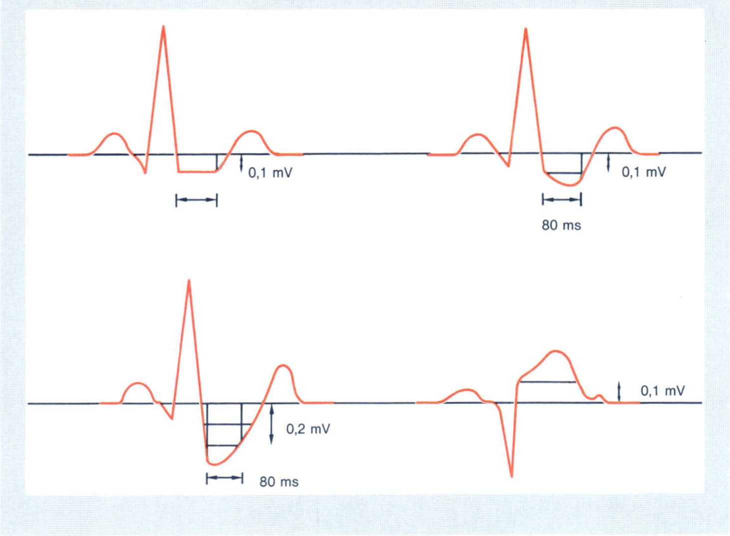

Fig. 23

Schematic drawing of the pathological alteration in the exercise ECG (by Rijneke and co-workers)

Predictive implications of the exercise ECG

False negative result of exercise ECG	Methodological reasons: Insufficient exercise intensity Insufficient ECG leads Missing typical clinical signs Incorrect interpretation by the physician Cardiac reason: Single vessel disease (in some cases) ECG alterations at rest: Right bundle branch block Left anterior hemiblock Right heart hypertrophy Drug induced changes: Beta-receptor blocking drugs (also nitrates, calcium antagonists and molsidomin prior to exercise testing) Quinidine Phenothiazine
False positive result of exercise ECG	ECG alterations at rest: Left bundle branch block, left heart hypertrophy WPW and LGL syndrome ST segment depression at rest more than 0.05 mV Drug induced changes: Digitalis Diuretics Antiarrhythmic drugs Tricyclic antidepressants α-methyldopa Other diseases: Mitral valve prolapse Hyperventilation Hypokalaemia Hypothyroidism Severe anaemia

Severe tachycardia at rest
Cardiomyopathy (congestive, hypertrophic)
Aortic valvular disease
Arterial hypertension

Criteria for test termination

Symptoms:
Dizziness, ataxia, progressive
anginal progressive dyspnoea

Findings:
ECG abnormalities
Progressive arrhythmias
Couplets, runs, ventricular tachycardias
Increasing number of supraventricular premature beats, atrial tachycardias, atrial flutter. New onset of atrial fibrillation

Progressive **conduction disturbances**
Widening of the QRS complex. New left bundle branch block

Progressive **repolarisation abnormalities**
(Increasing ST segment depression)
Horizontal depression more than 0.2 mV
progressive ST segment elevation
elevation of ST segment (discontinuation in any case)

Haemodynamic abnormalities:
Progressive fall in blood pressure
Failure of blood pressure to rise (less than 10 mmHg per exercise step)
Excessive blood pressure rise
($\geq$250 mmHg systolic
$\geq$120 mmHg diastolic).

ECG examples

Example of severe right heart overload (17-year-old girl, cor pulmonale due to mucoviscidosis). ECG vertical axis, right bundle branch block, disturbances of repolarization in the right heart leads, pronounced S up to V_6 indicating right chamber overload.

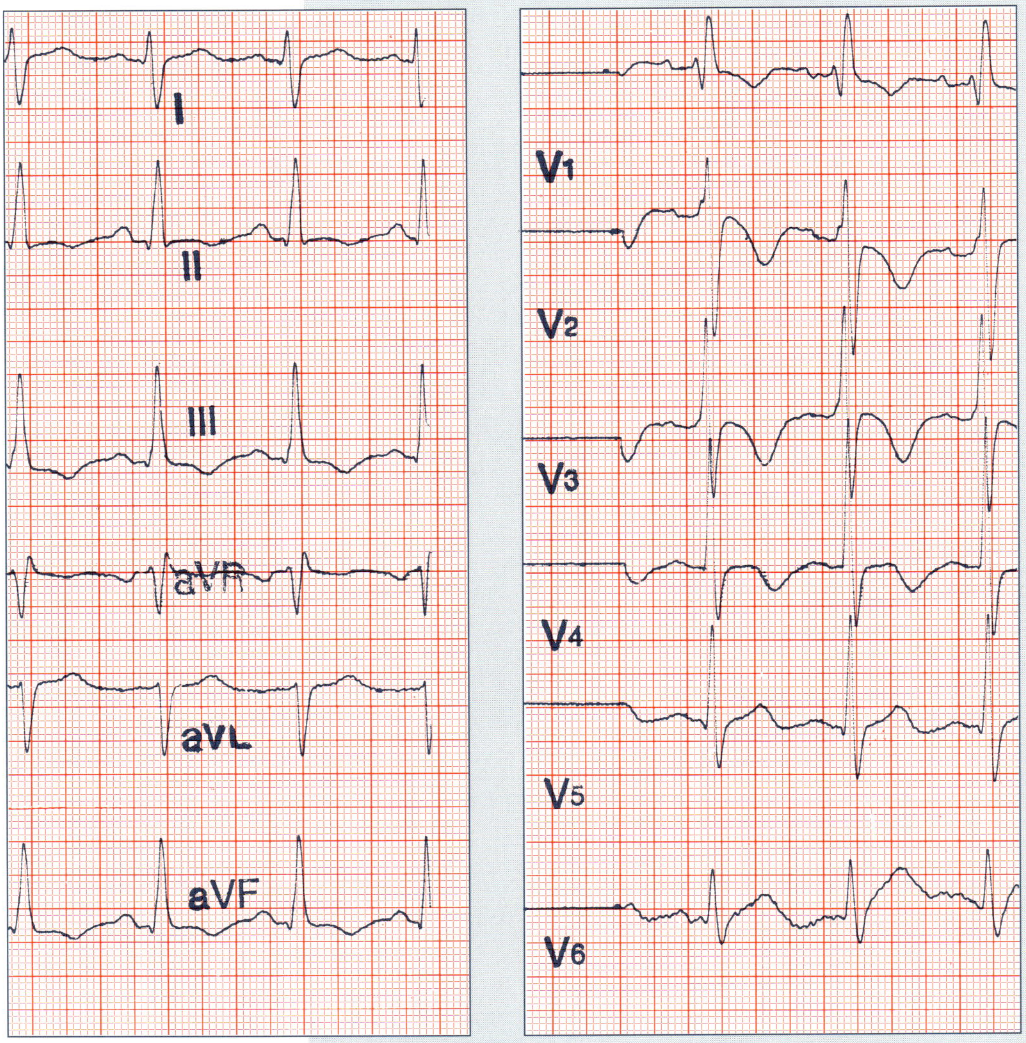

Example of left ventricular hypertrophy due to aortic insufficiency. Left axis deviation, deep S waves in V_3 and V_4, high R amplitudes in the left precordial leads, pronounced repolarization abnormalities due to left heart hypertrophy.

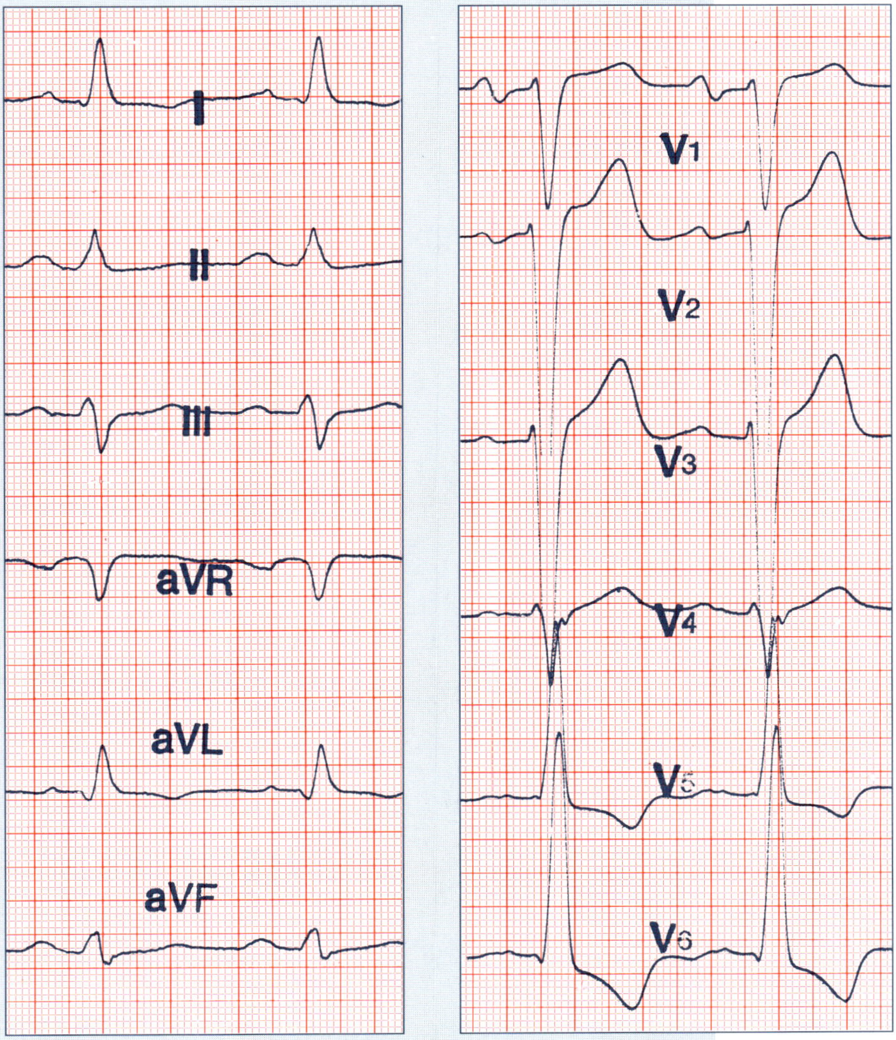

Typical findings of acute inferior myocardial infarction with a strictly posterior infarction and extension to the lateral wall. The first ECG shows ST elevation in the inferior leads, ST segment depression in V_2 (indicating the posterior position) and ST elevation in V_5 and V_6.

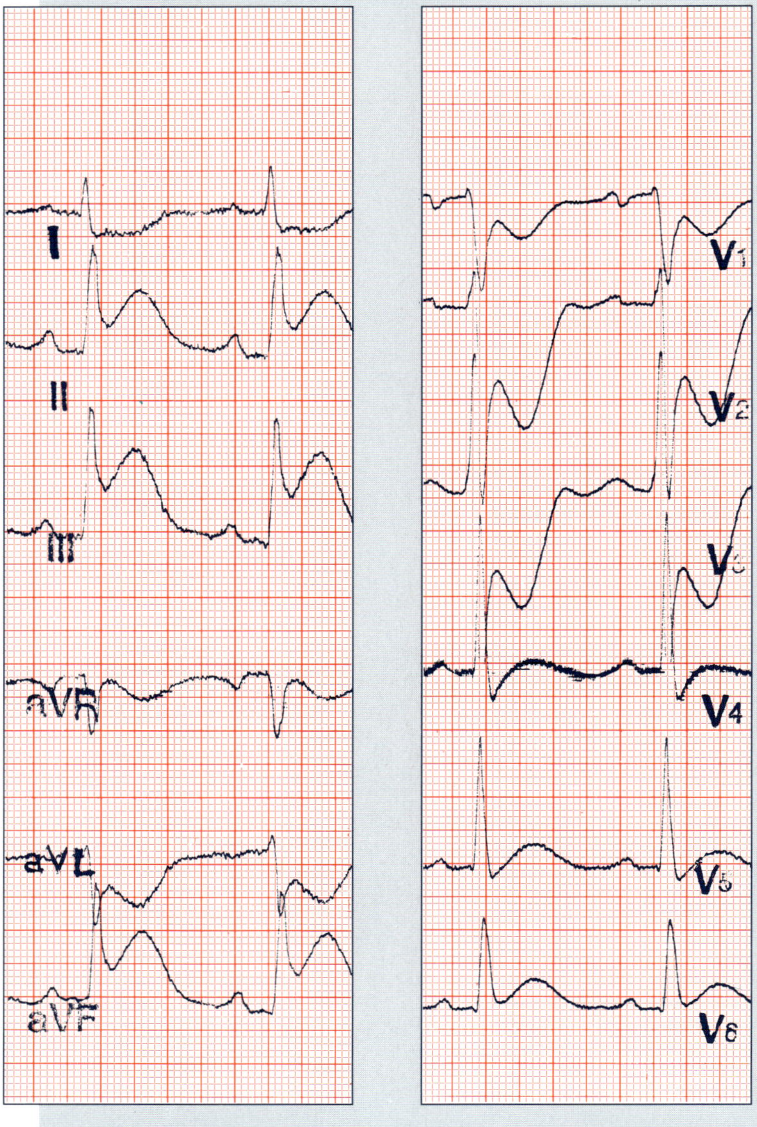

One day after the acute MI there are Q waves and loss of R amplitude. The ST segment depression in the right precordial leads is less pronounced.

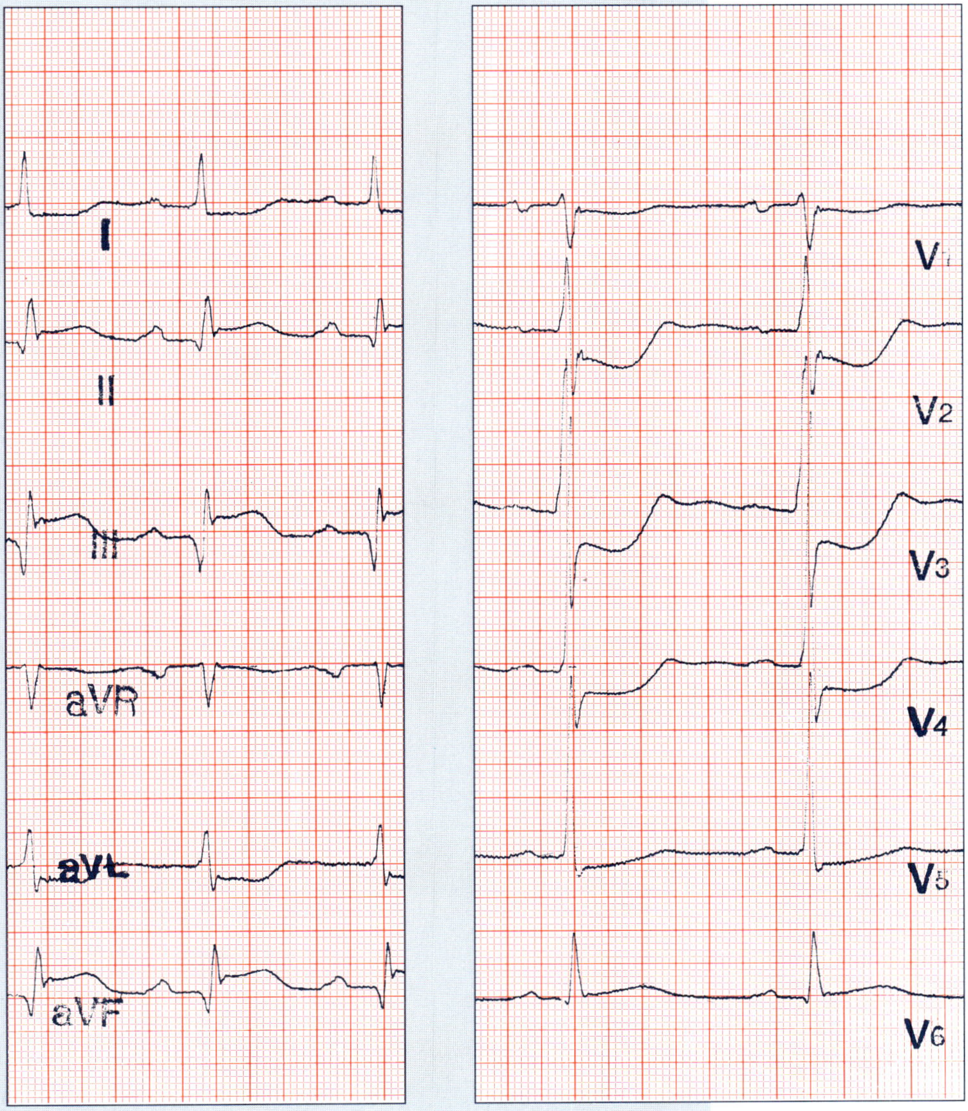

Typical finding of non-specific repolarization abnormalities as a normal variant. Woman, 25 years old, without cardiac disease. T waves normalize during exercise testing. No structural heart disease.

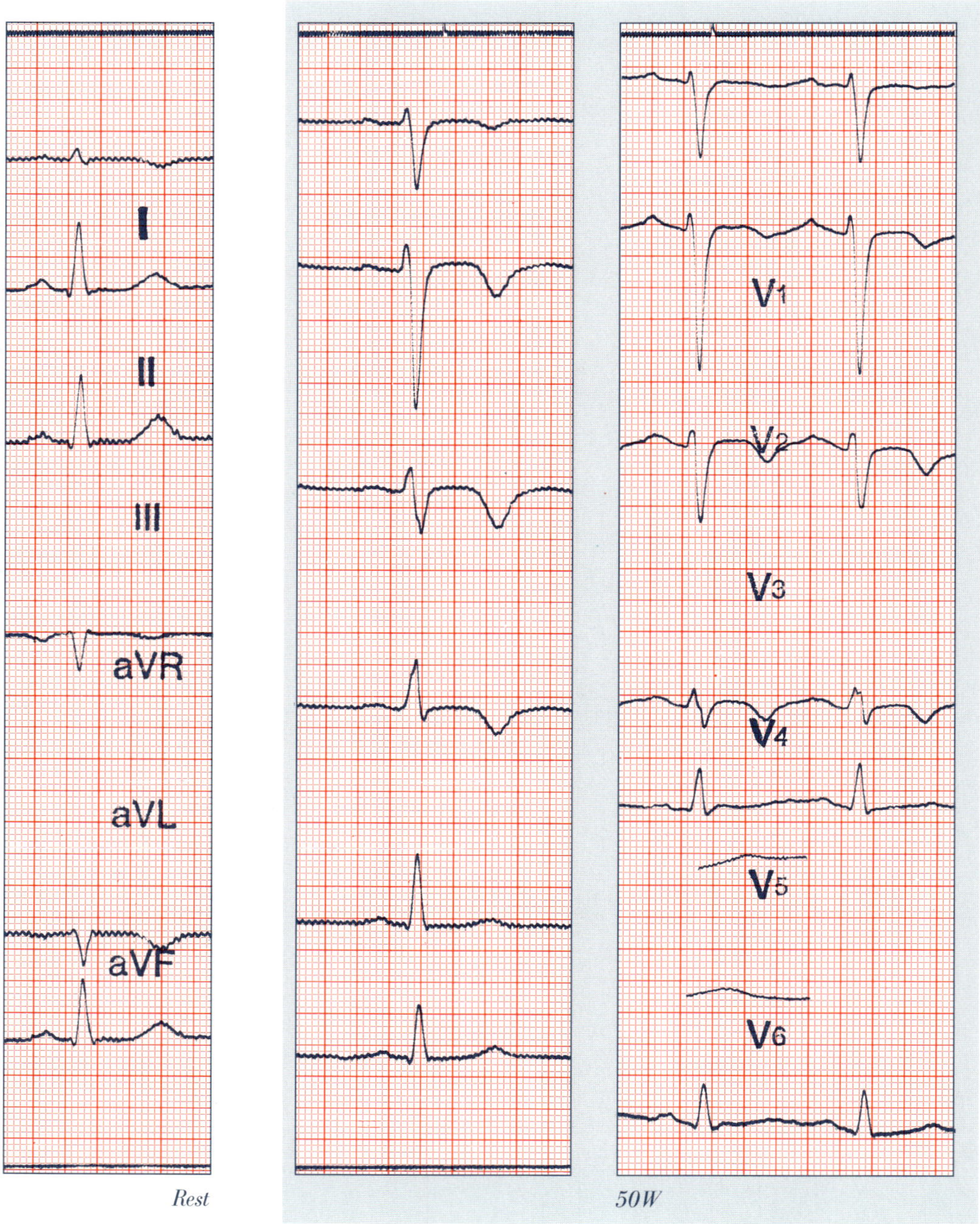

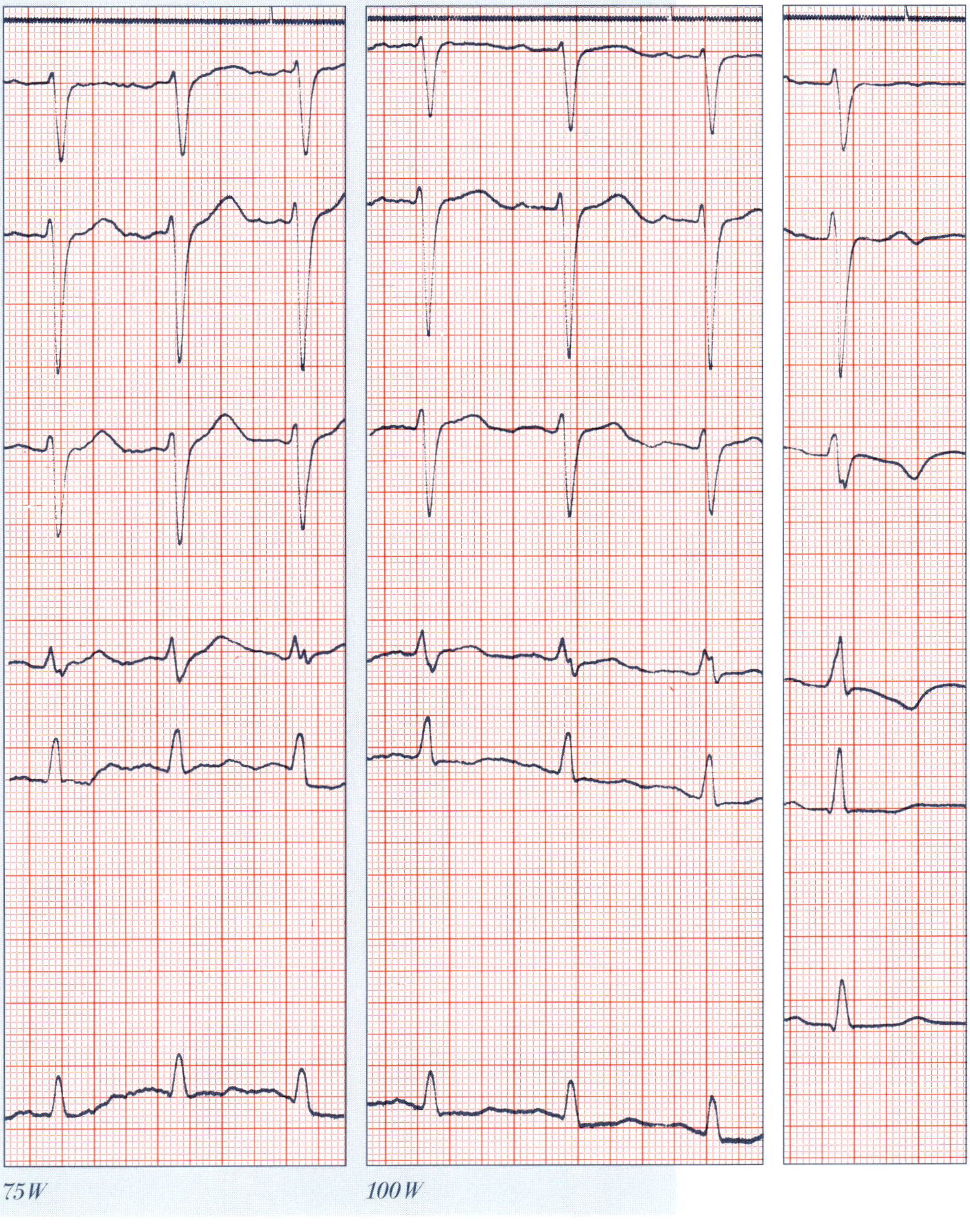

75 W *100 W*

Repolarization abnormalities in a young male patient with acute myocarditis (biopsy proven). One day later the ECG was normal and no structural heart disease was observed.

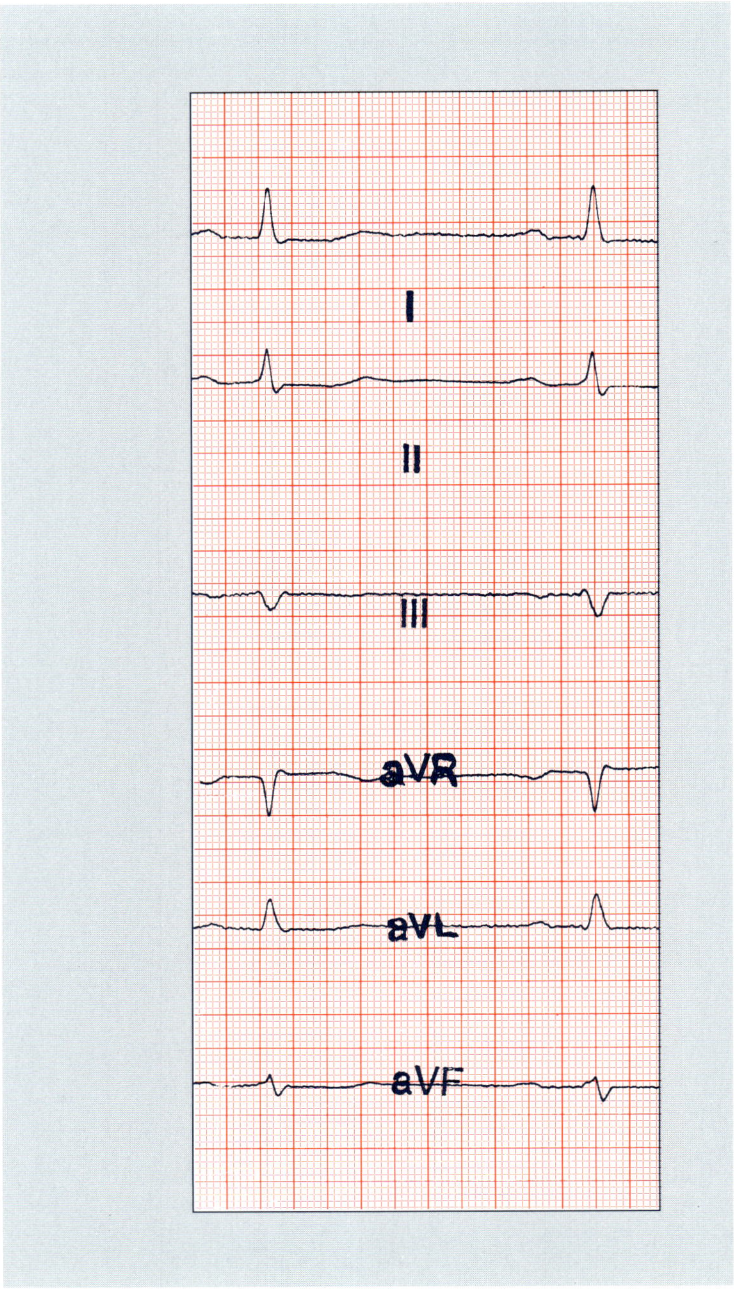

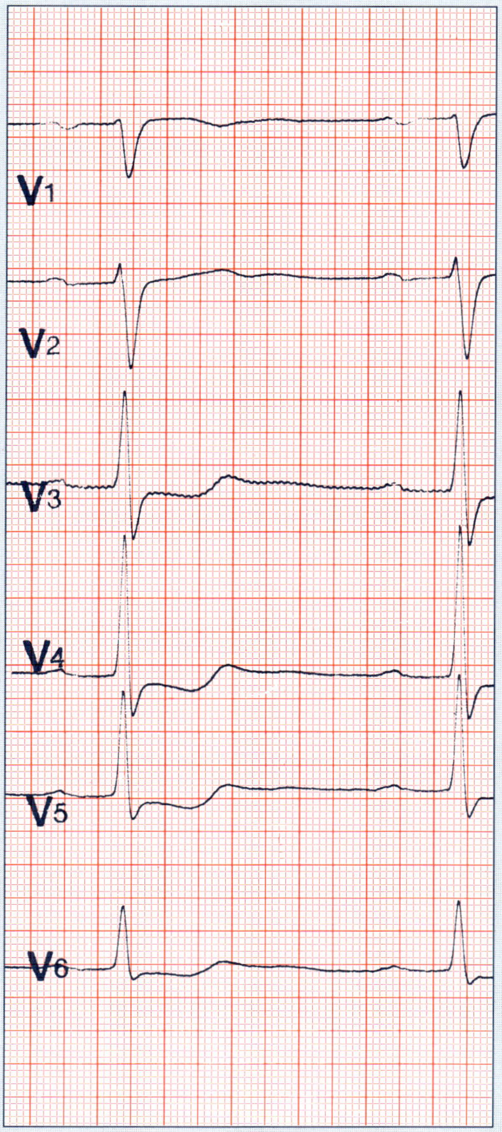
V1
V2
V3
V4
V5
V6

Woman, 58 years old, with acute haemorrhage in the subarachnoidal space. Non-specific repolarization abnormalities with ST segment elevation in the anteroseptal leads due to

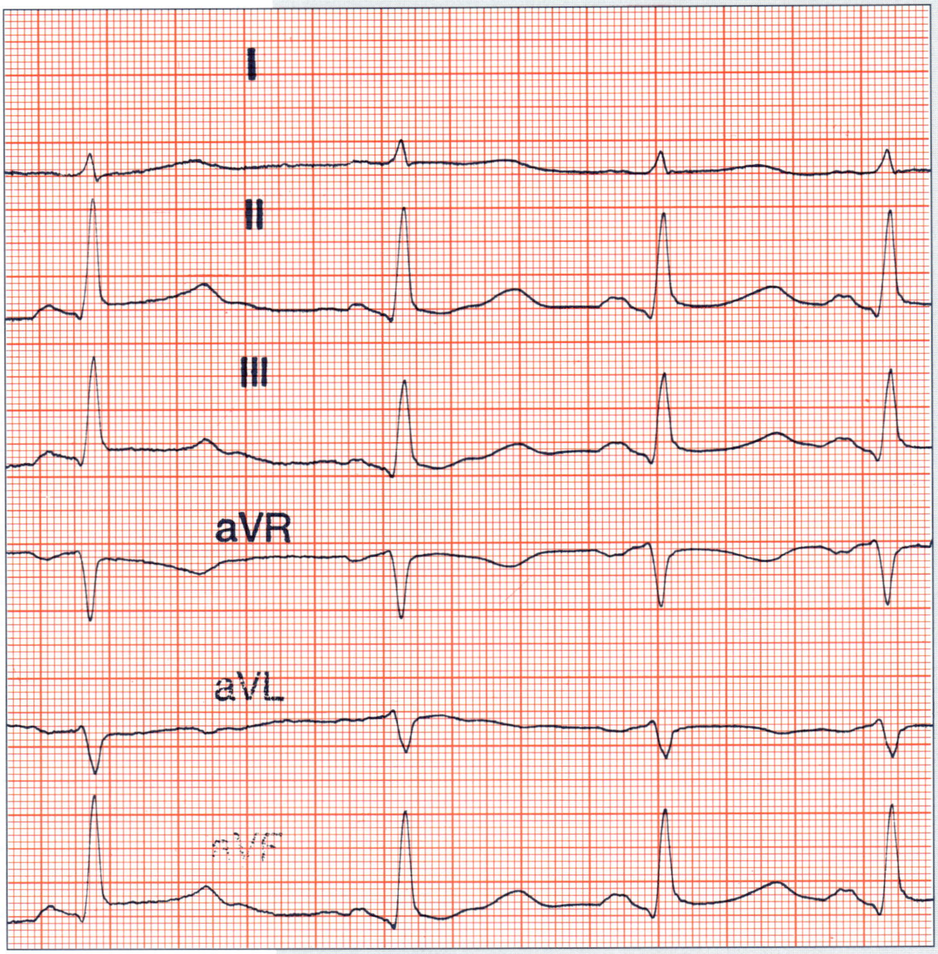

an increase of intracranial pressure. Normal values for heart-specific enzymes (CK and CKMB), pronounced prolongation for QT interval (0.46 s or 130 %).

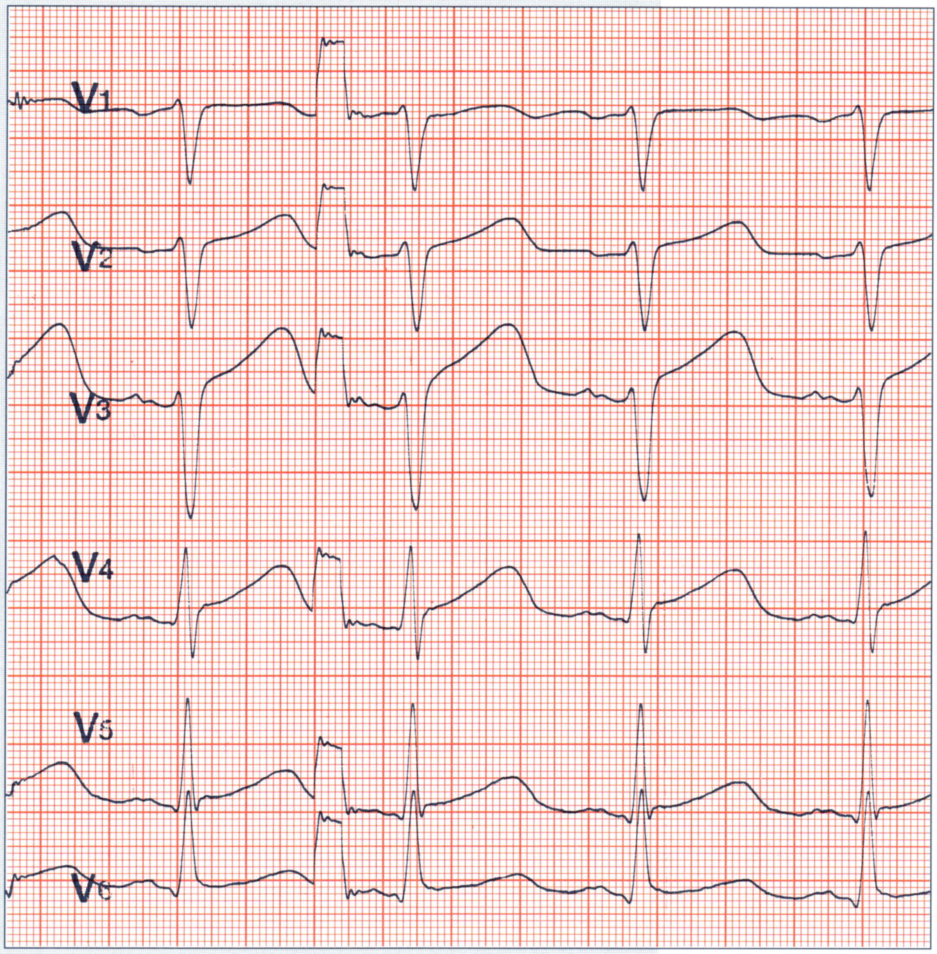

Pronounced abnormalities of repolarization and depolarization due to accidental intoxication with potassium containing drugs and simultaneously renal insufficiency with chronic dialysis. Serum potassium: 8.6 mval/l.

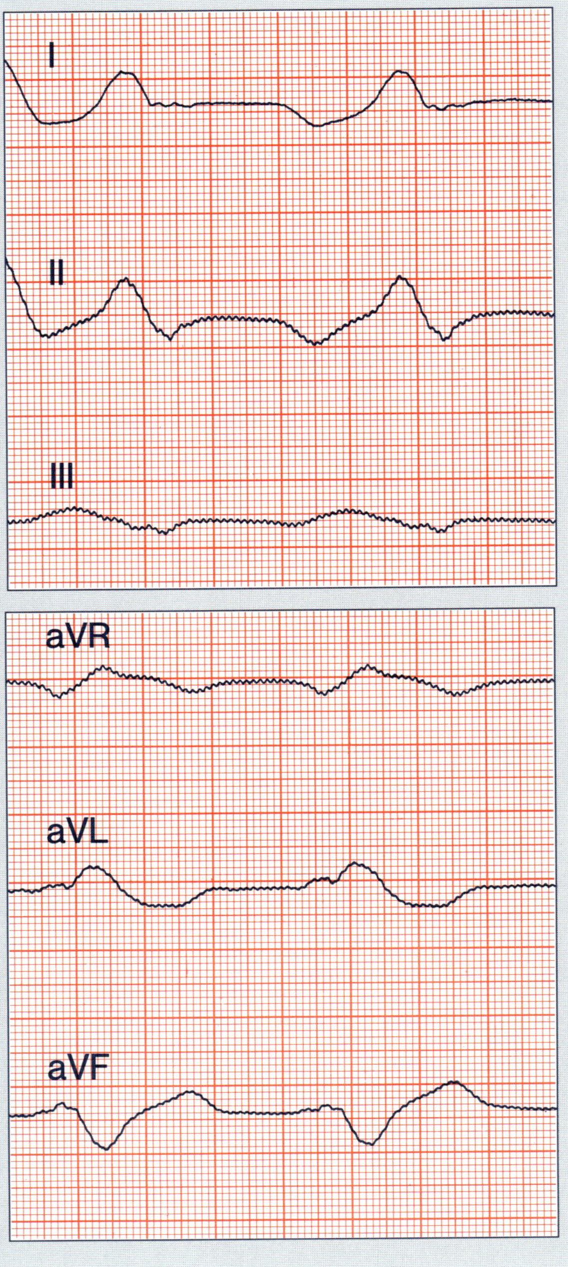

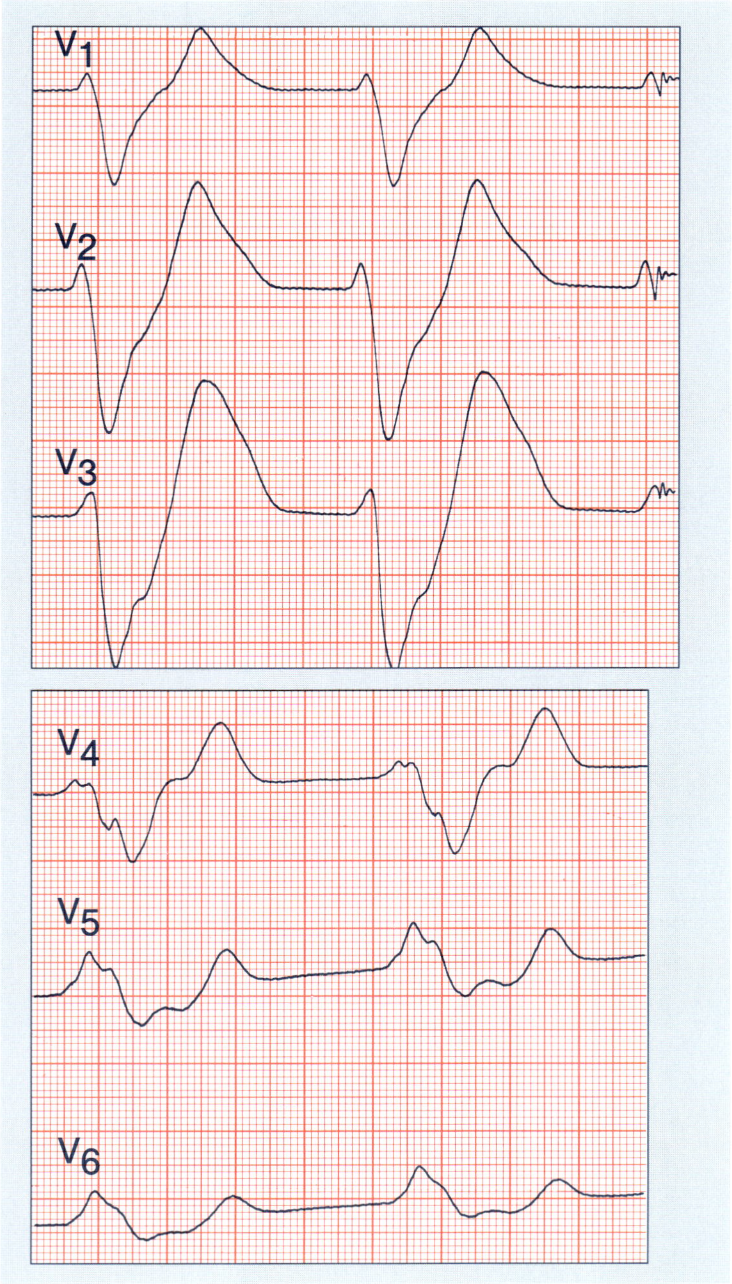
V1
V2
V3
V4
V5
V6

ECG in a young female with pseudo-Bartter's syndrome and renal potassium wasting leading to extremely low potassium values. Initially potassium was 2.25mval/l, heart rate 80/min and QT interval 0.53s or 160%.

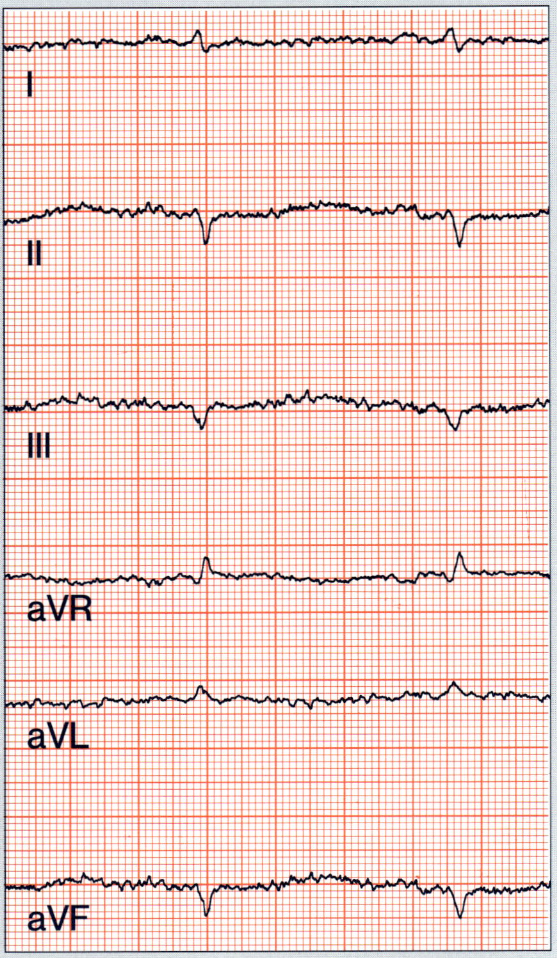

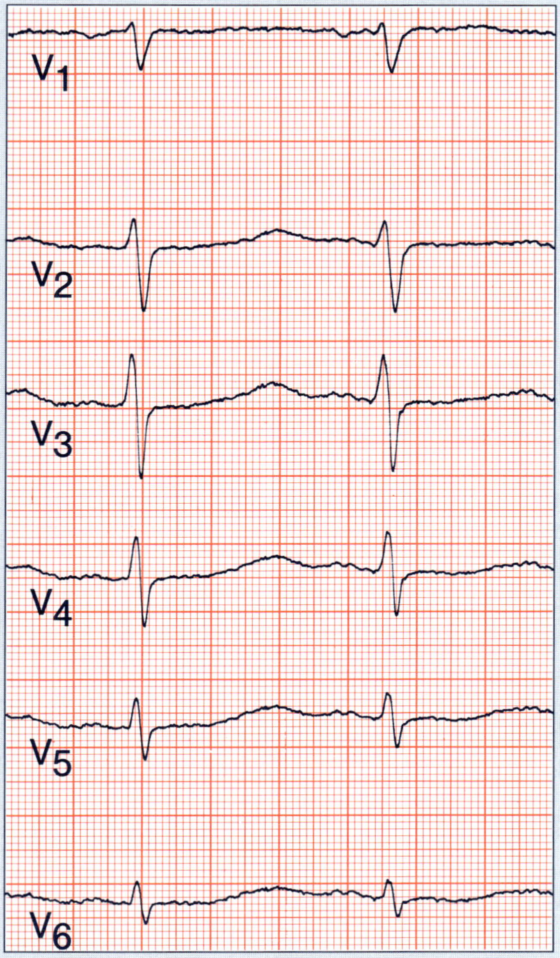
V1
V2
V3
V4
V5
V6

56-year-old woman with idiopathic intermittent atrial fibrillation and atrial flutter. Spontaneous sinus rhythm during therapy with propafenone. Sudden end of the tachycardia with sinus node arrest due to overdrive suppression.

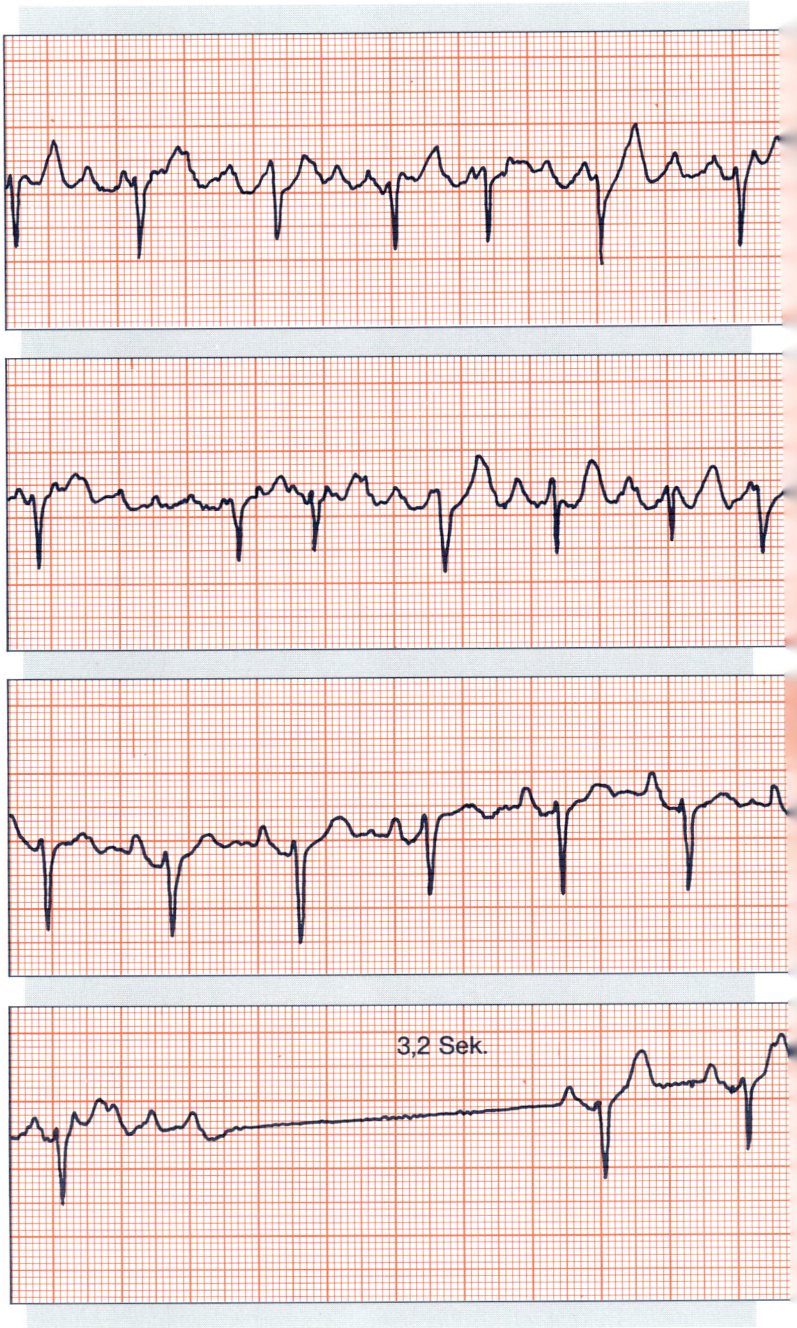

The sinus node function has been suppressed by overstimulation. The final rhythm is sinus rhythm with supraventriclar extrasystoles.

ECG continued

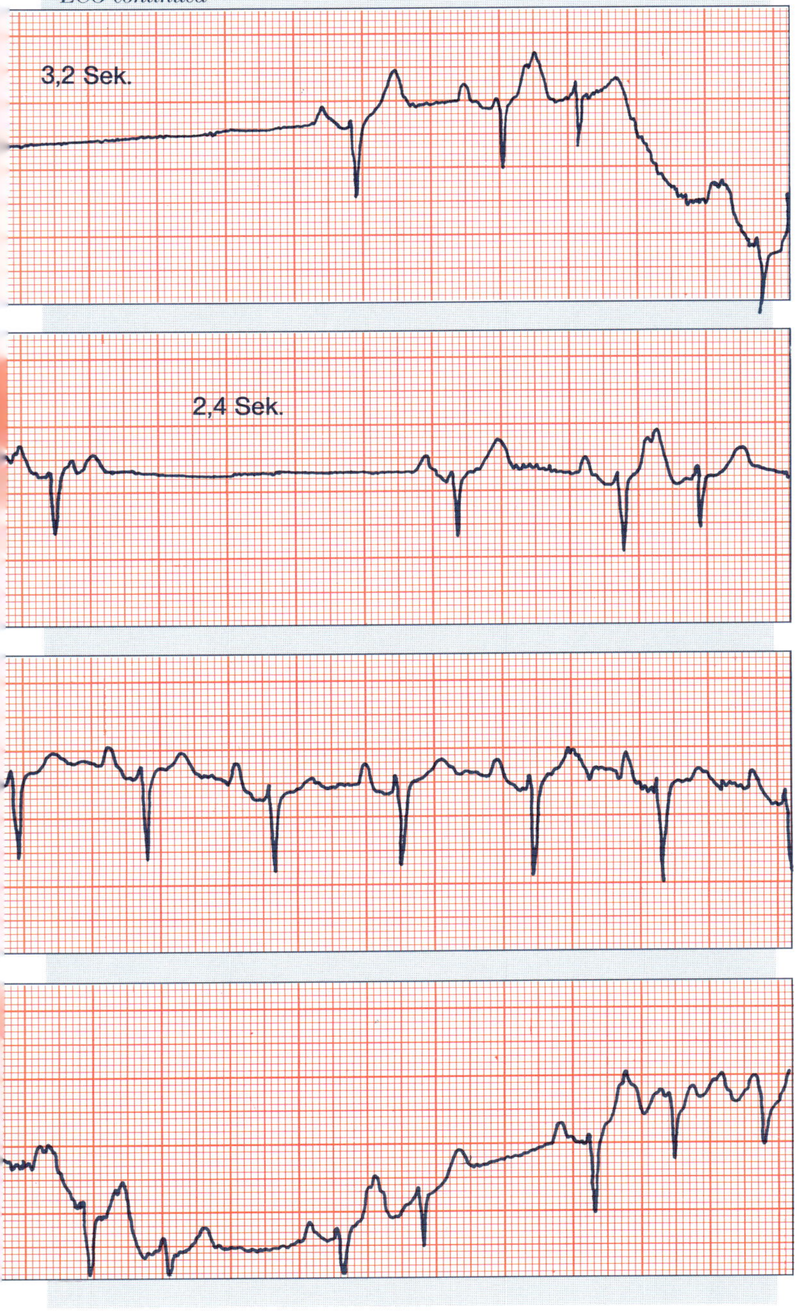

Exercise-induced AV block II° with sudden reduction of exercise tolerance and clinical symptoms. Finding was reproducible.

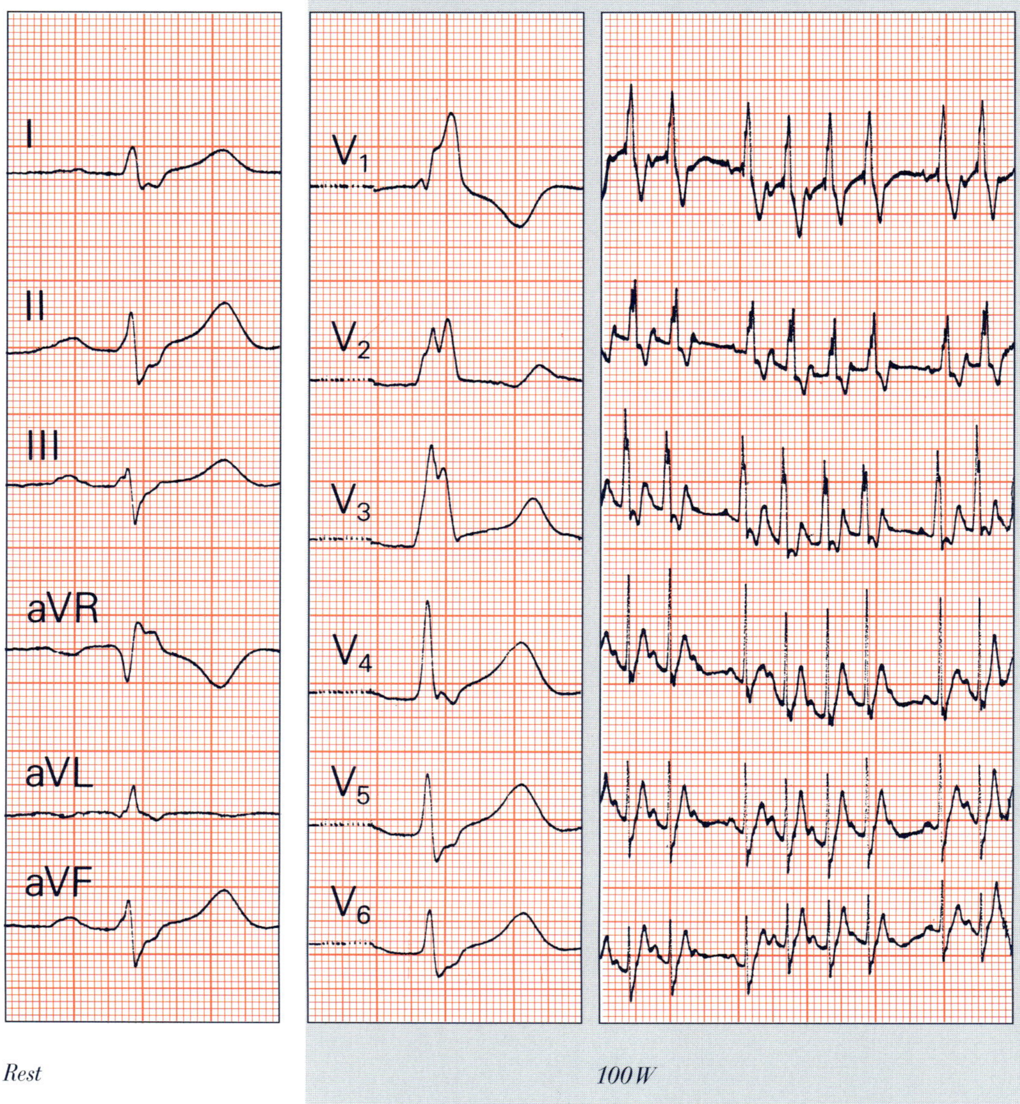

Rest

100 W

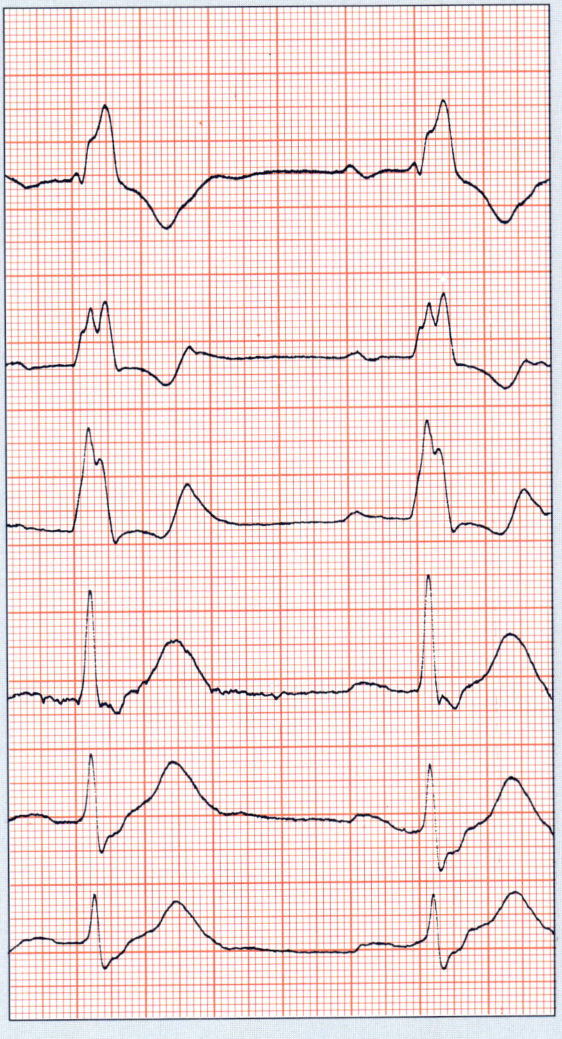

100 W

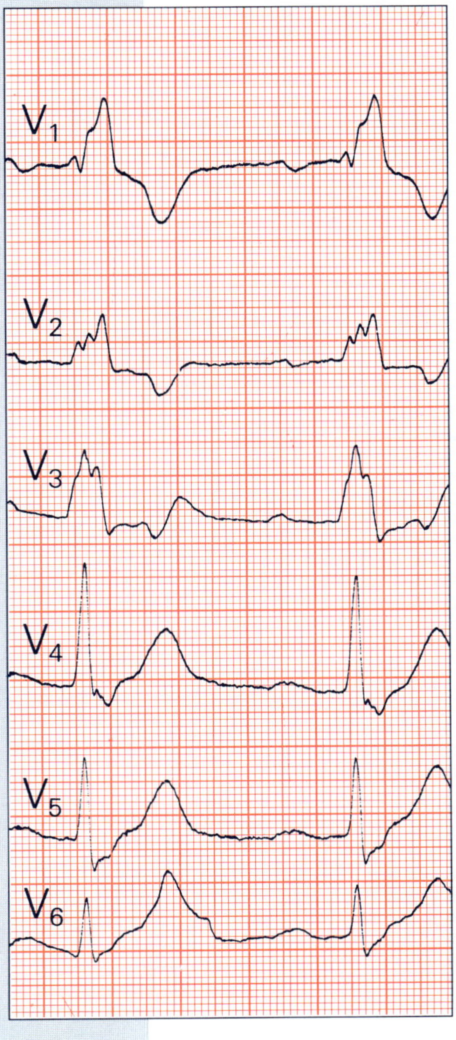

150 W

Same patient as in previous figure (page 82/83) after implantation of a pacemaker (2-chamber system, DDD-system). During pacemaker therapy normal physical capacity, no symptoms. The etiology remained unsolved. Lyme disease was not proven.

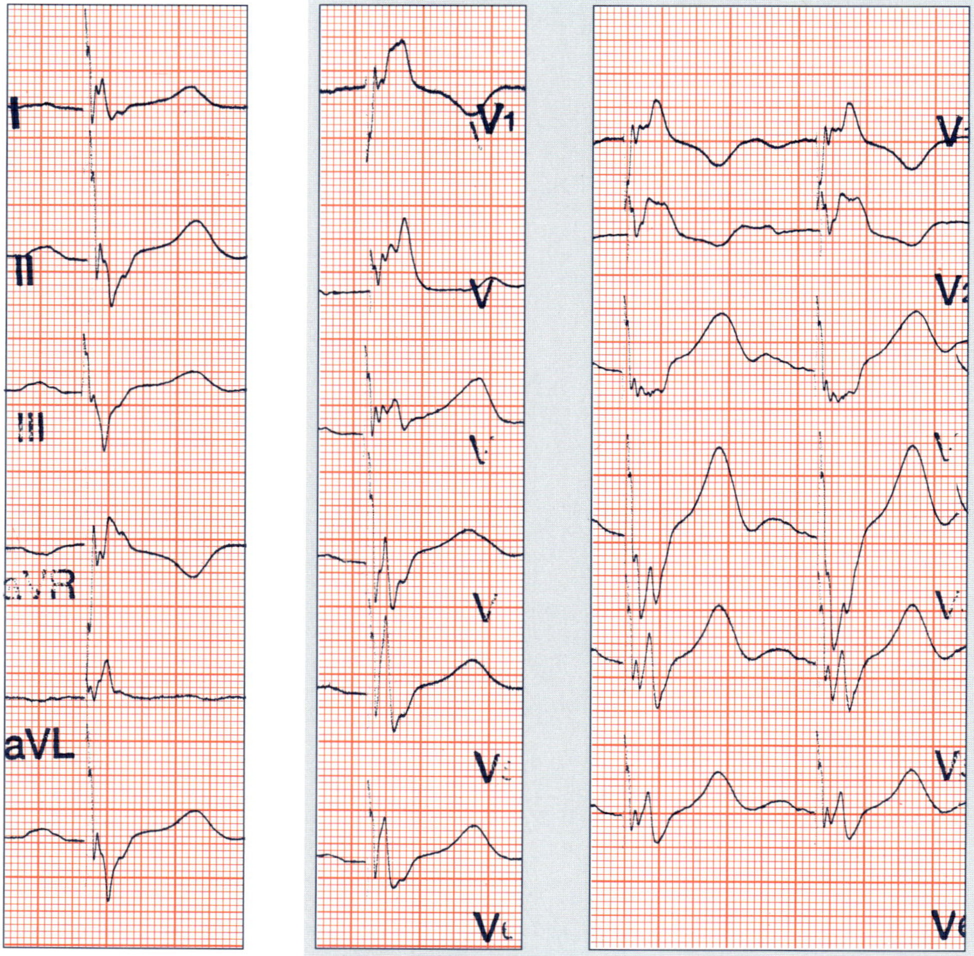

Rest

75W

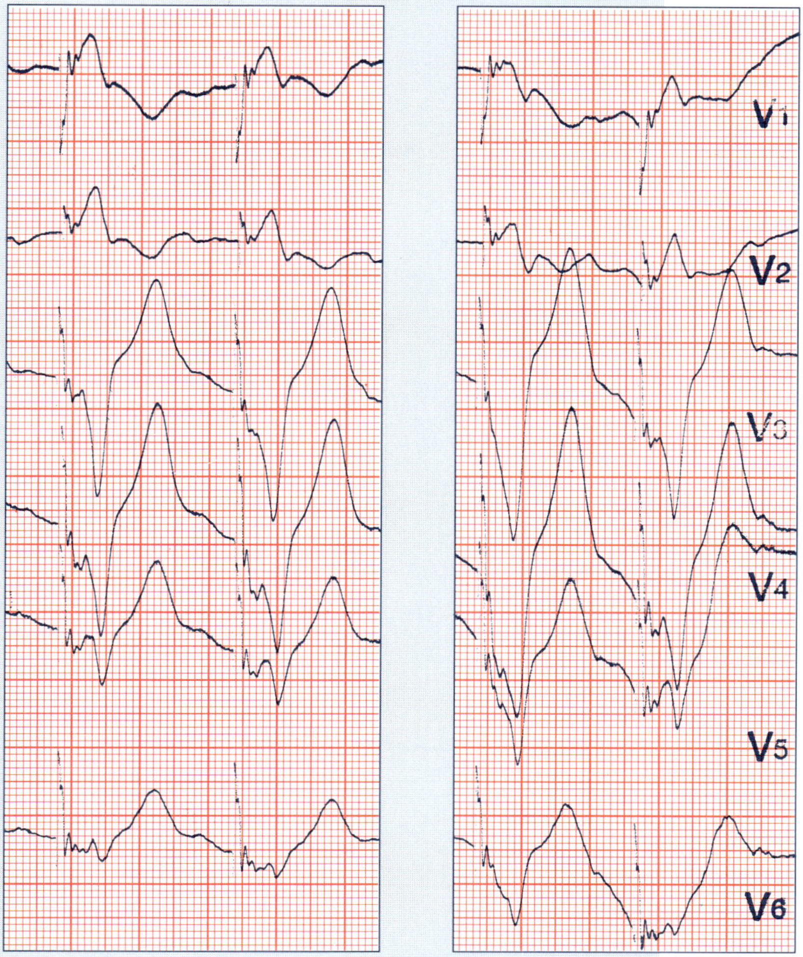

125 W *150 W*

Patient with changing symptoms: days with reduced physical capacity, days with normal exercise capacity. Ambulatory ECG shows intermittent AV block II°.

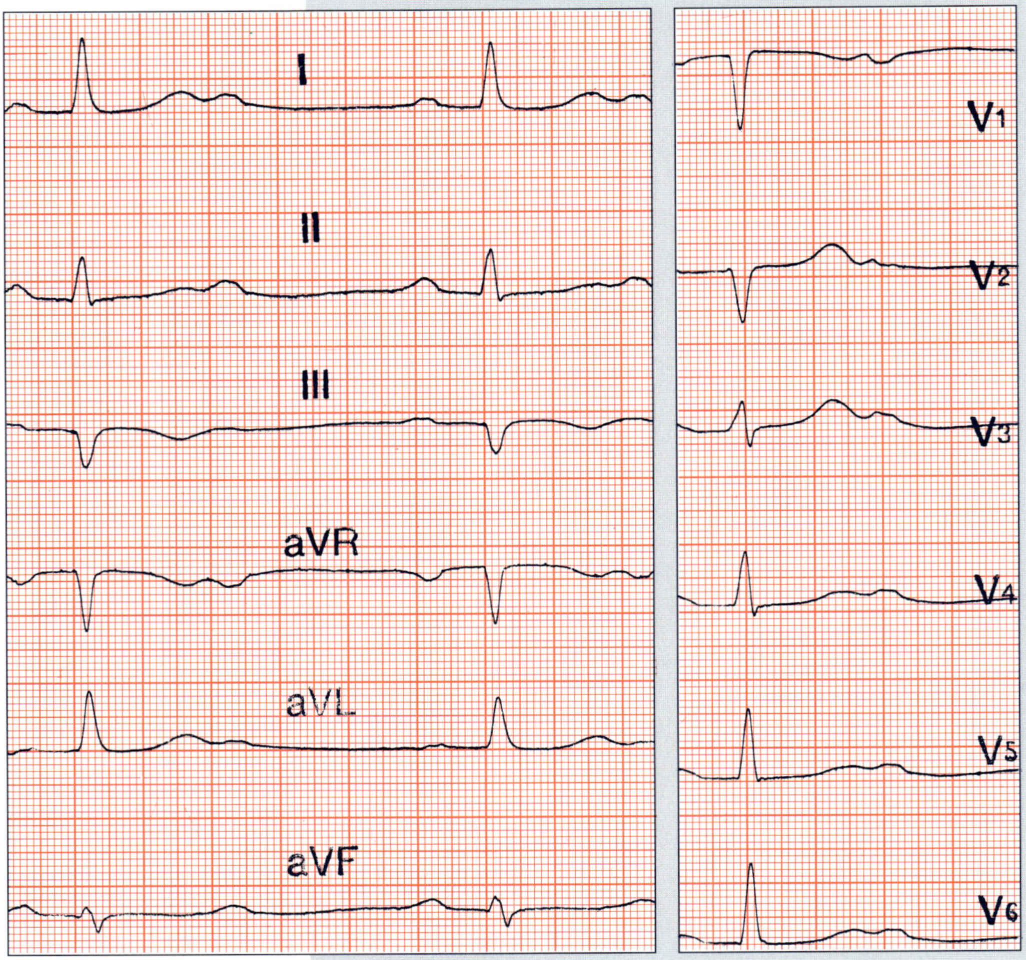

After implantation of a pacemaker (2-chamber system) symptoms disappeared and resulted in good exercise tolerance. Etiology unknown.

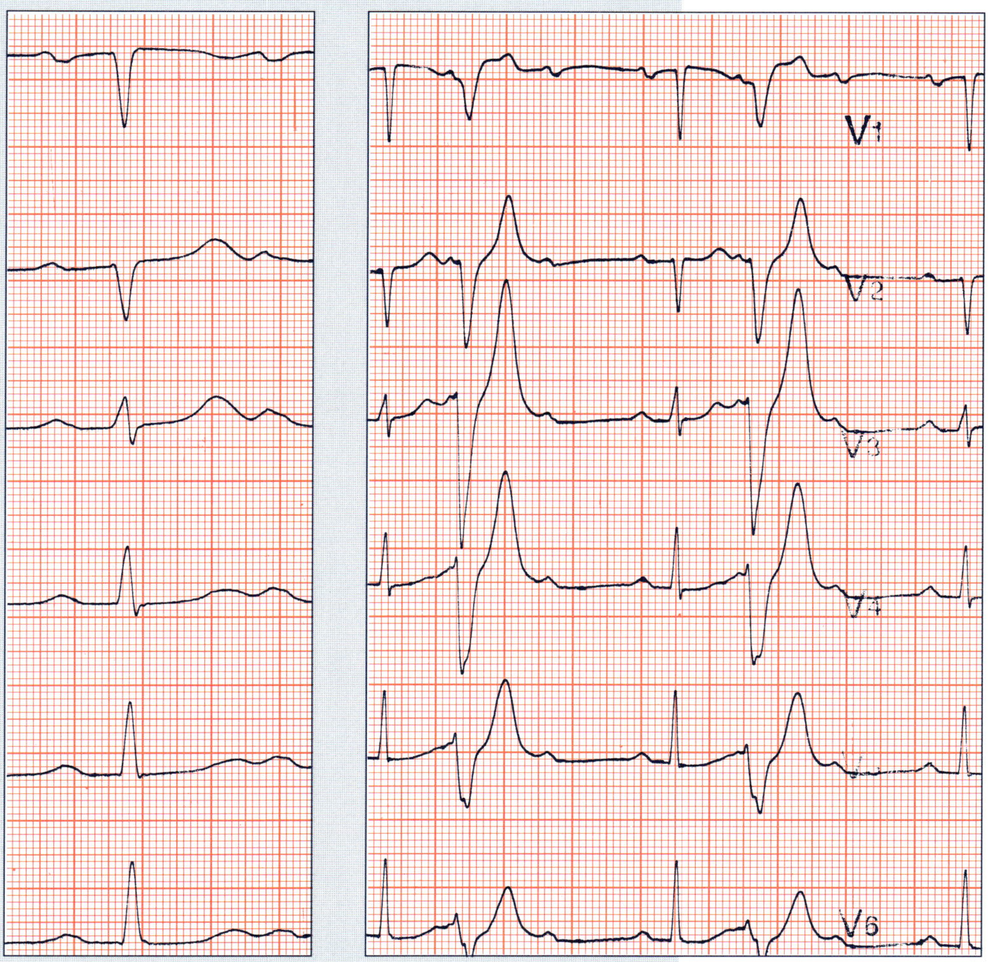

78-year-old male with syncope. The ECG shows total AV block (complete heart block). The underlying disease was CAD with an old inferior MI combined with strictly posterior and lateral ischaemia.

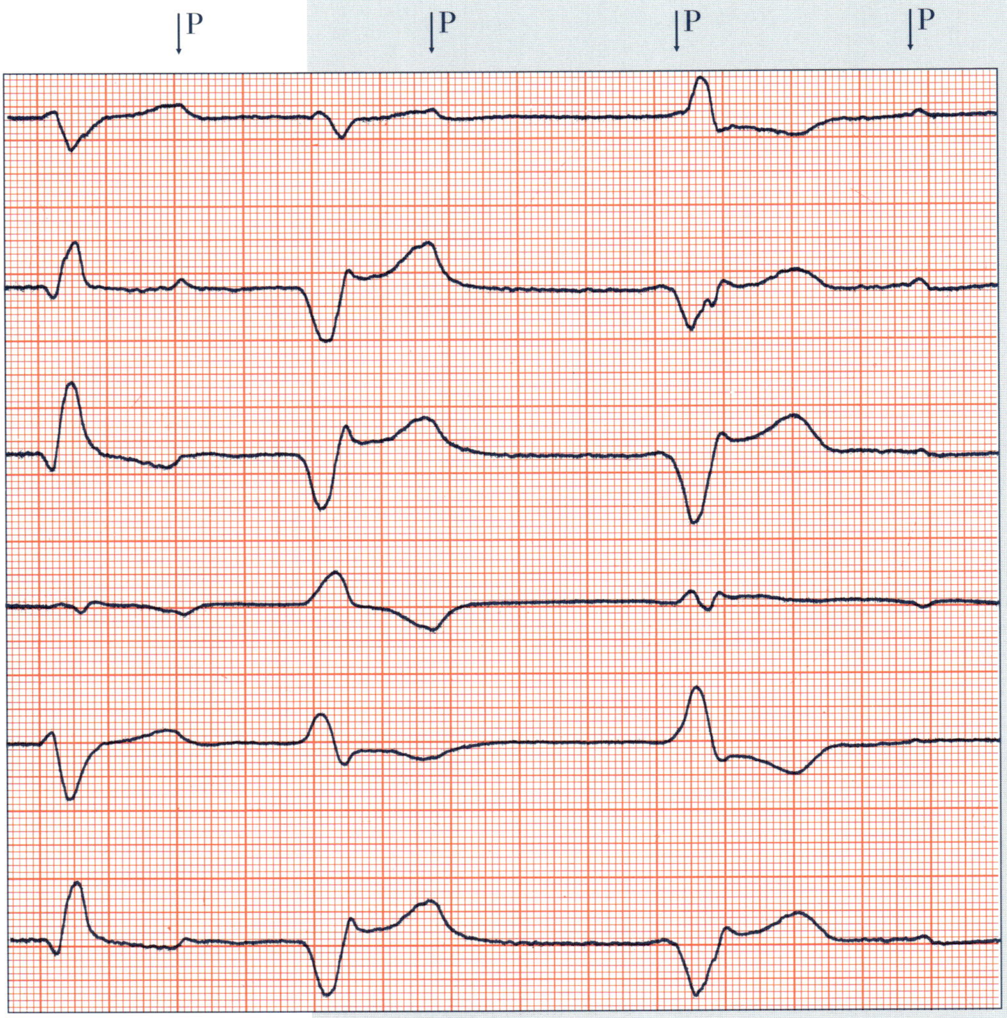

P waves are marked by arrows and the next figures (pages 90 and 91) show the ECG after implantation of a 2-chamber pacemaker system (DDD-system).

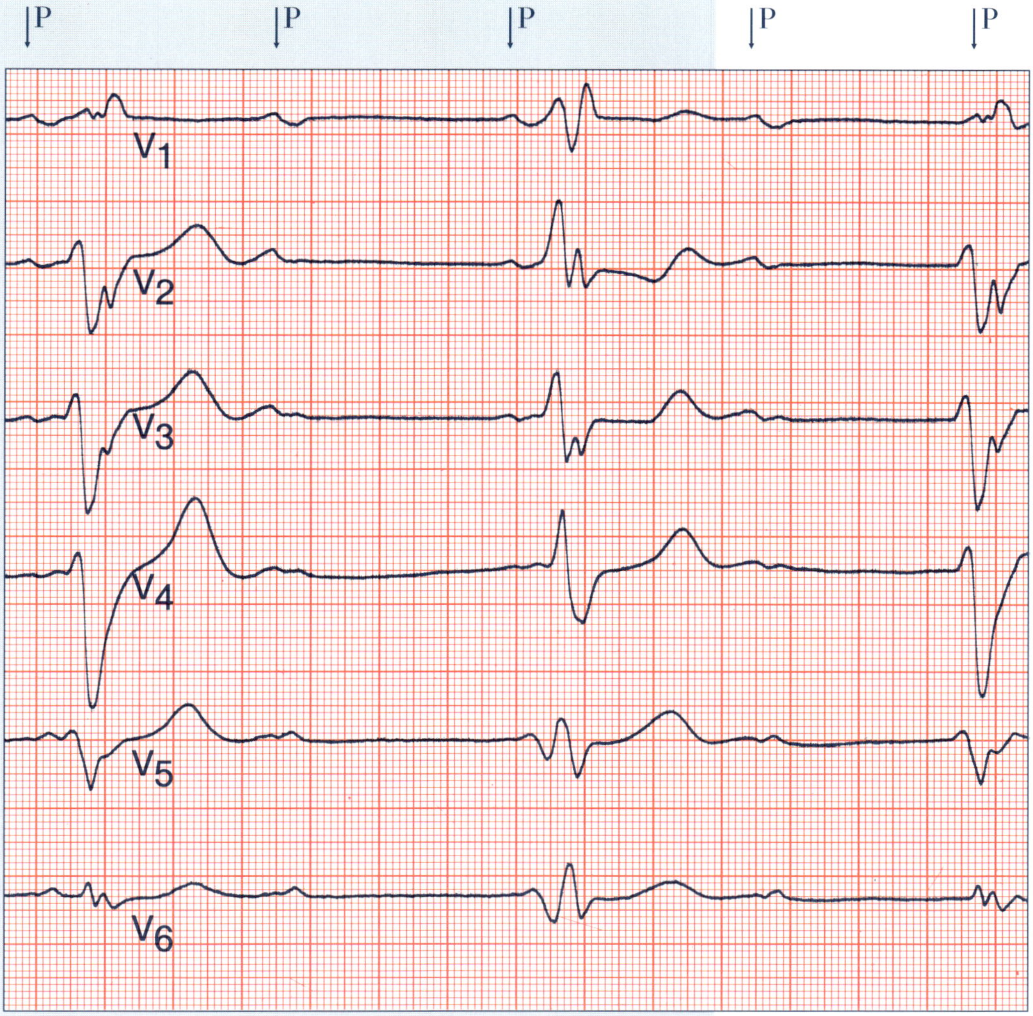

Same patient as in previous figure (page 88) after implantation of a pacemaker (2-chamber system).

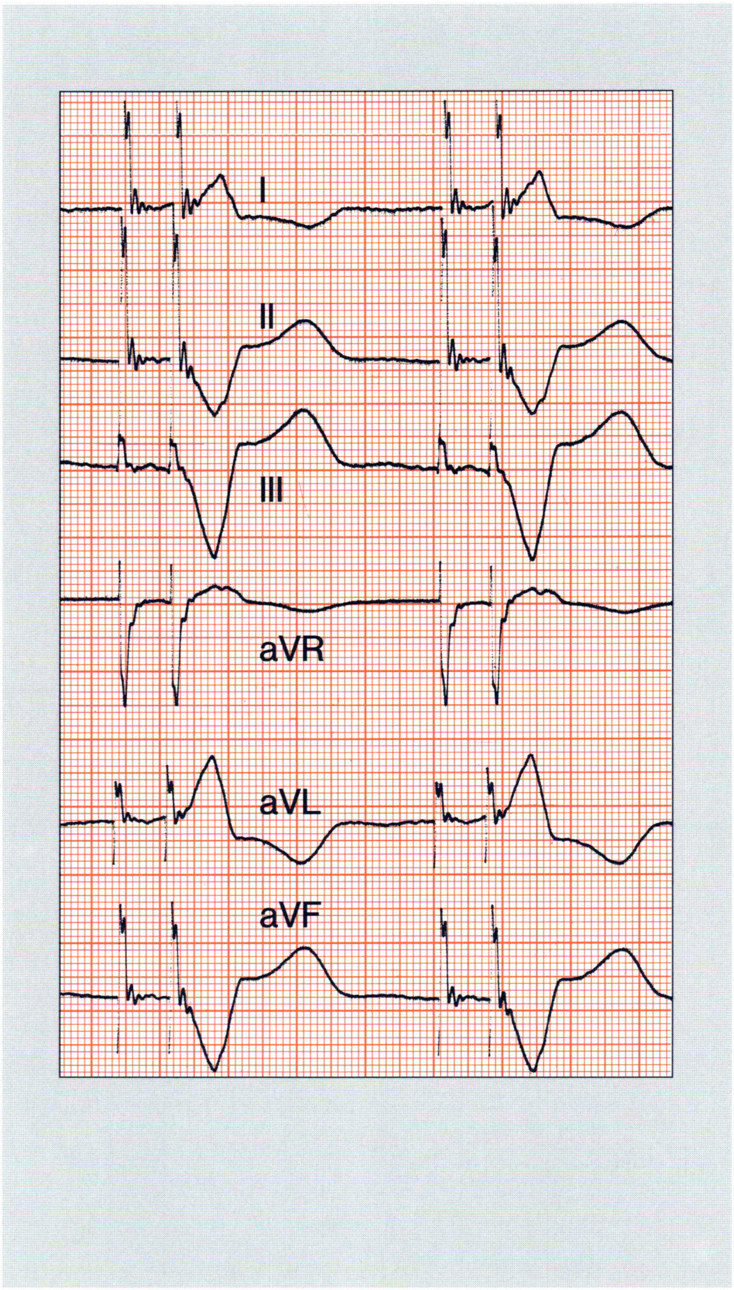

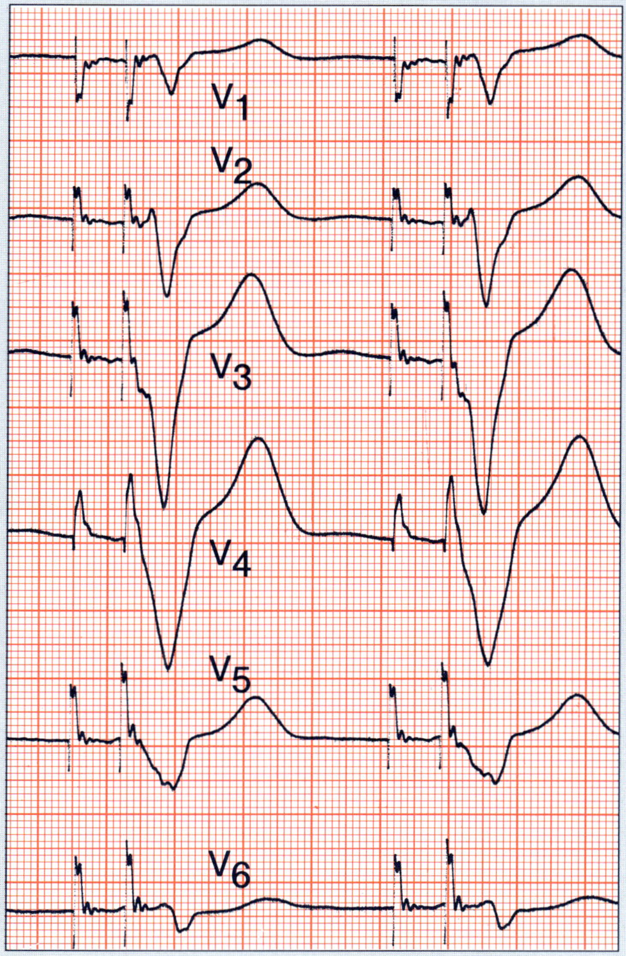
V_1
V_2
V_3
V_4
V_5
V_6

56-year-old patient after coronary bypass surgery. P waves without fixed connection to the following QRS complex indicating a typical finding of AV dissociation.

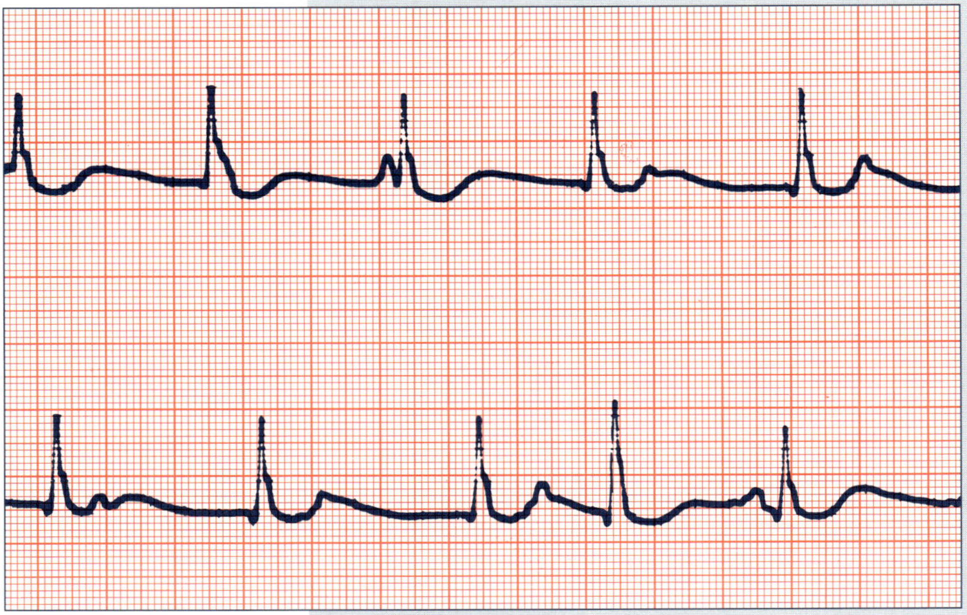

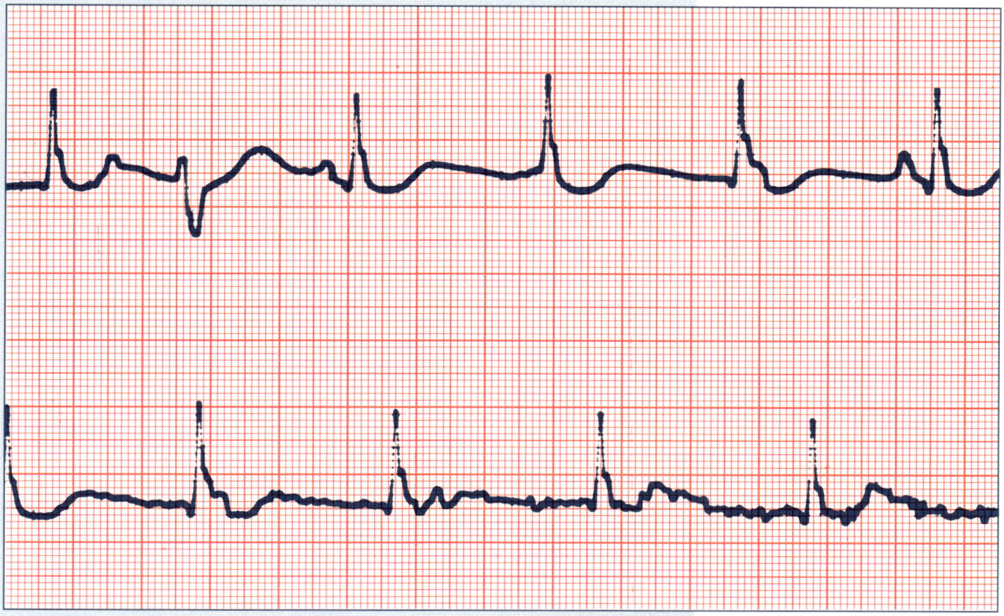

Typical example of a 2-chamber pacemaker system. The pacemaker has been programmed to a single-chamber stimulation (VVI) because of intermittent atrial flutter and fibrillation. After sinus rhythm following drug therapy there was an AV block and the exercise tolerance was markedly reduced.

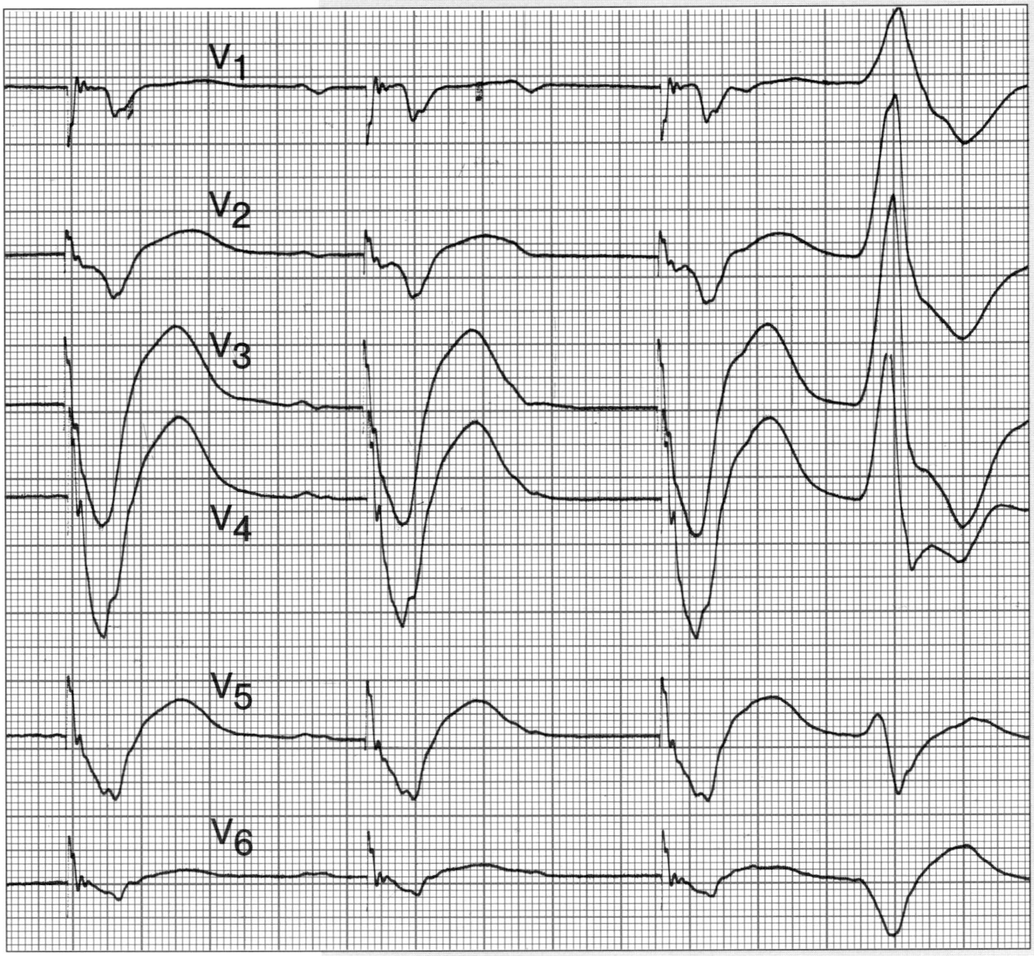

The pacemaker was then programmed to a 2-chamber stimulation (DDD-mode). Correct sensing and stimulation can be seen in the figure on page 96.

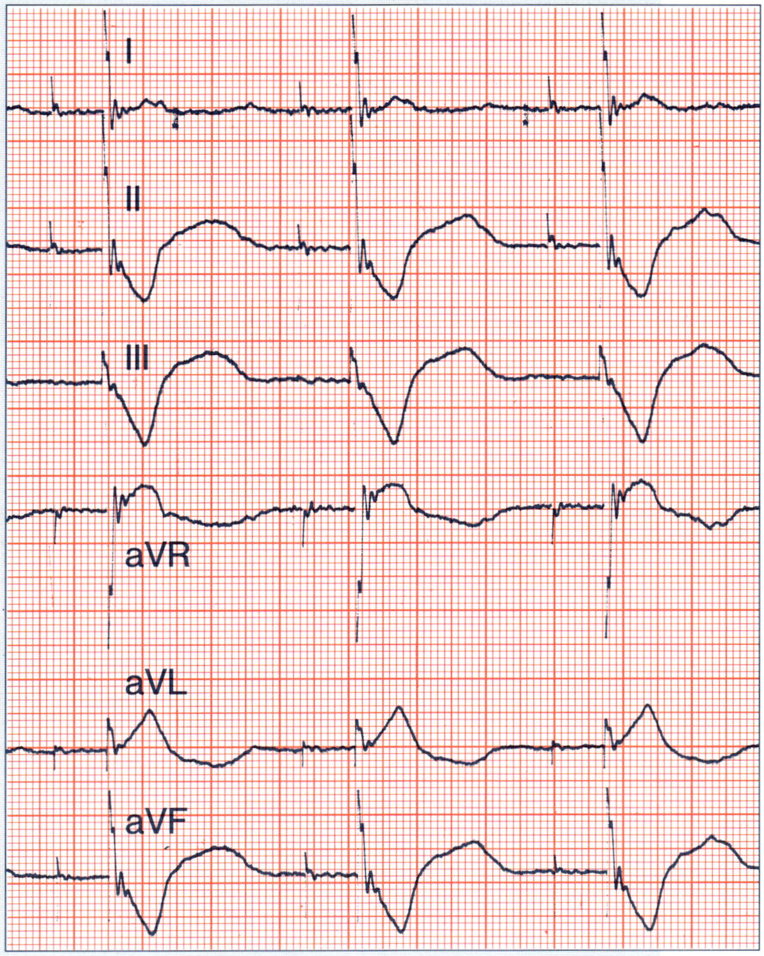

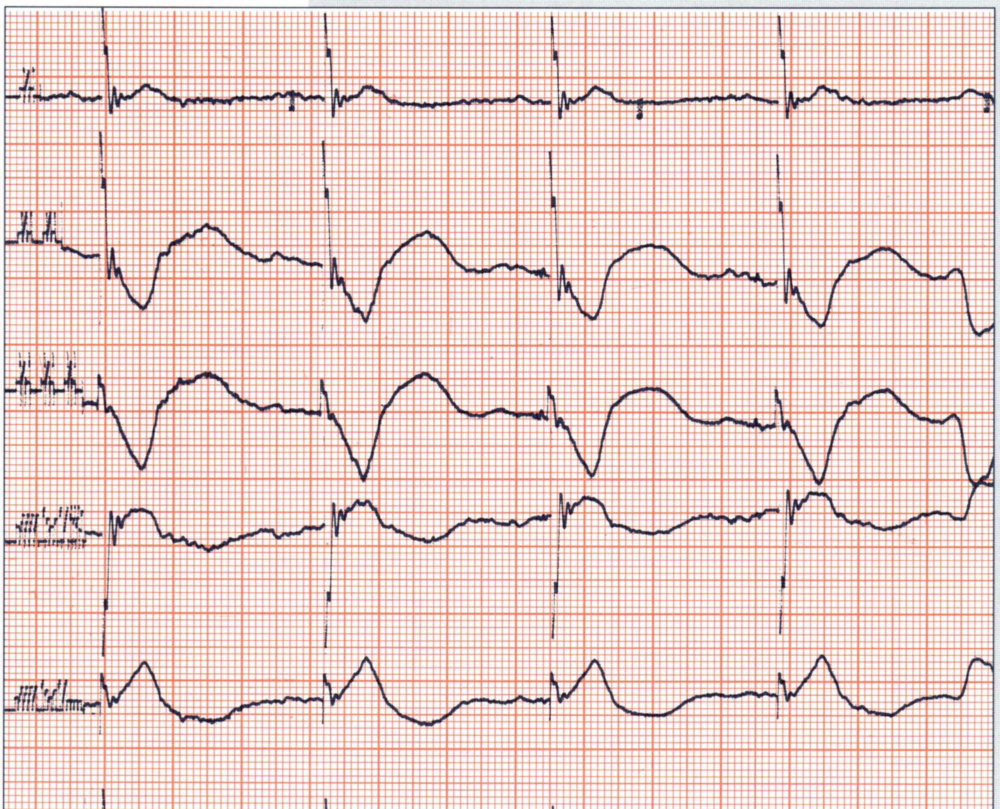

Patient, 77 years old, with coronary artery disease and syncope. The ECG shows intermittent supraventricular tachycardia (a), followed by sinus bradycardia. In addition, the recordings show silent ischaemic episodes (b). Pacemaker was inserted due to tachycardias requiring drug therapy with secondary symptomatic bradycardias.

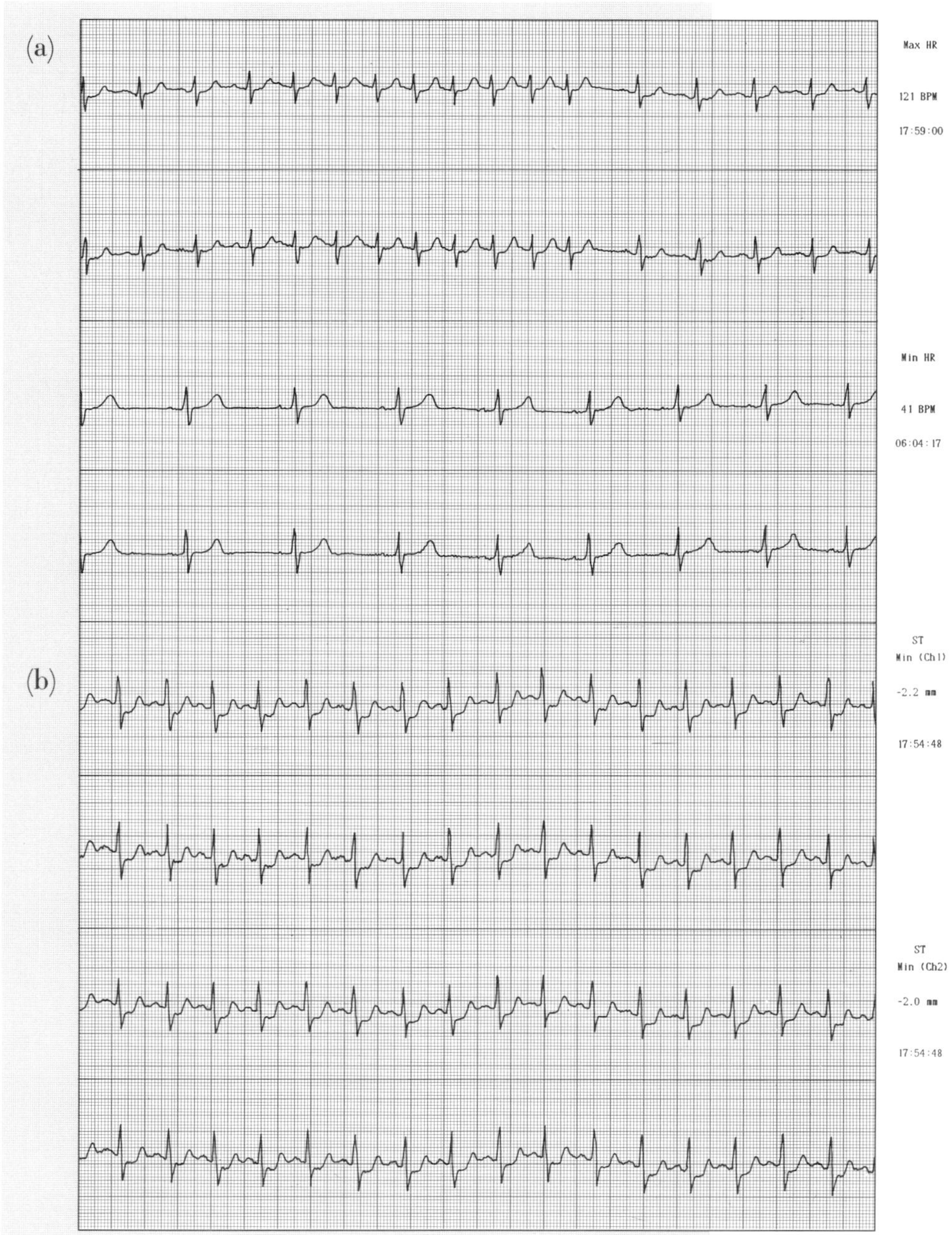

53-year-old patient engaged in endurance sports with intermittent atrial flutter (a). Invasive examination revealed no structural myocardial disease. Therapy was initiated by overstimulation with a burst (b) (800 impulses/min) converting atrial flutter to atrial fibrillation (c), followed by spontaneous sinus rhythm some minutes later (d). Drug therapy was then performed using verapamil and quinidine.

15:37:50

(a)

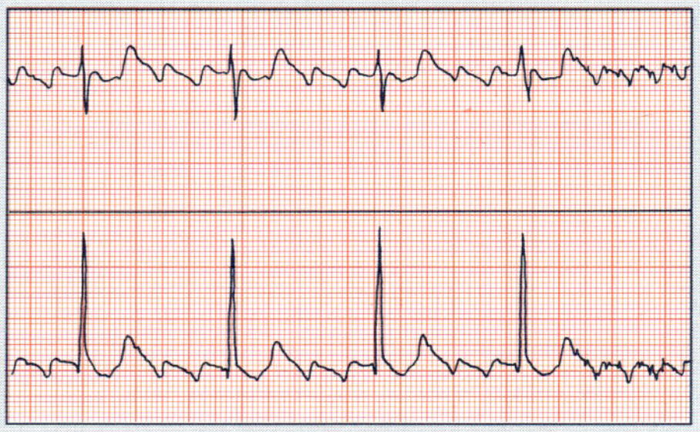

15:38:00

(b)

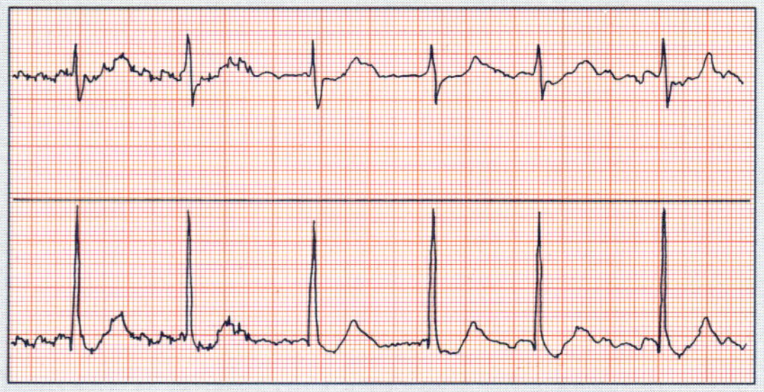

15:39:00

(c)

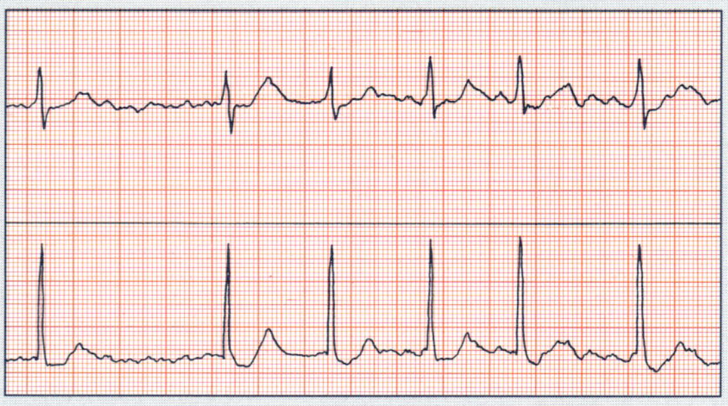

15:39:20

(d)

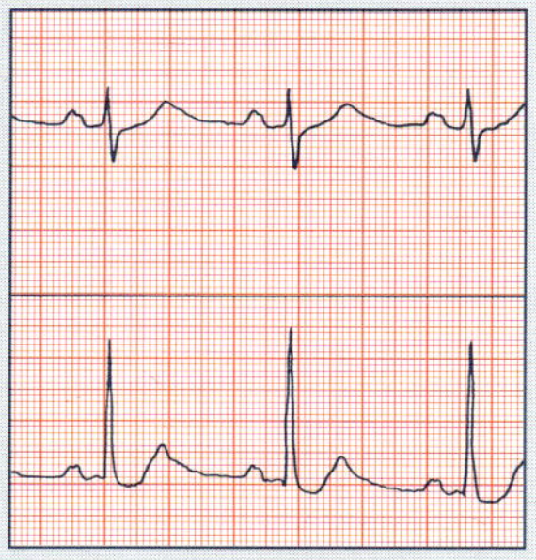

Same patient as on page 98.

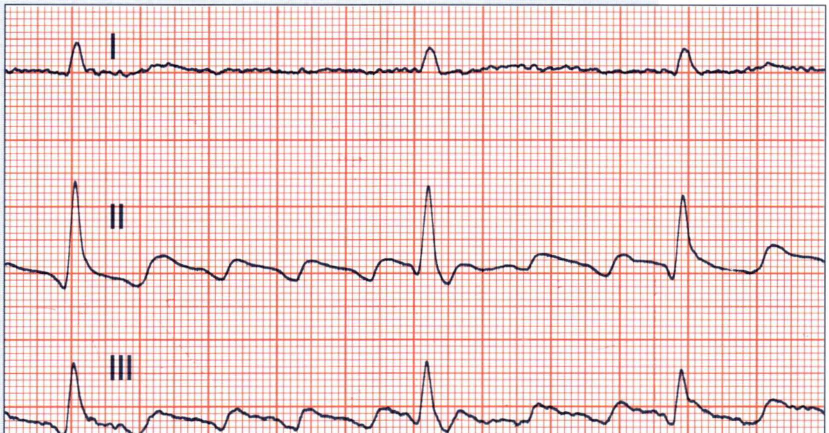

Same patient as on page 98. This figure shows normal ECG and the leads from intracardial ECG from the right atrium (page 103).

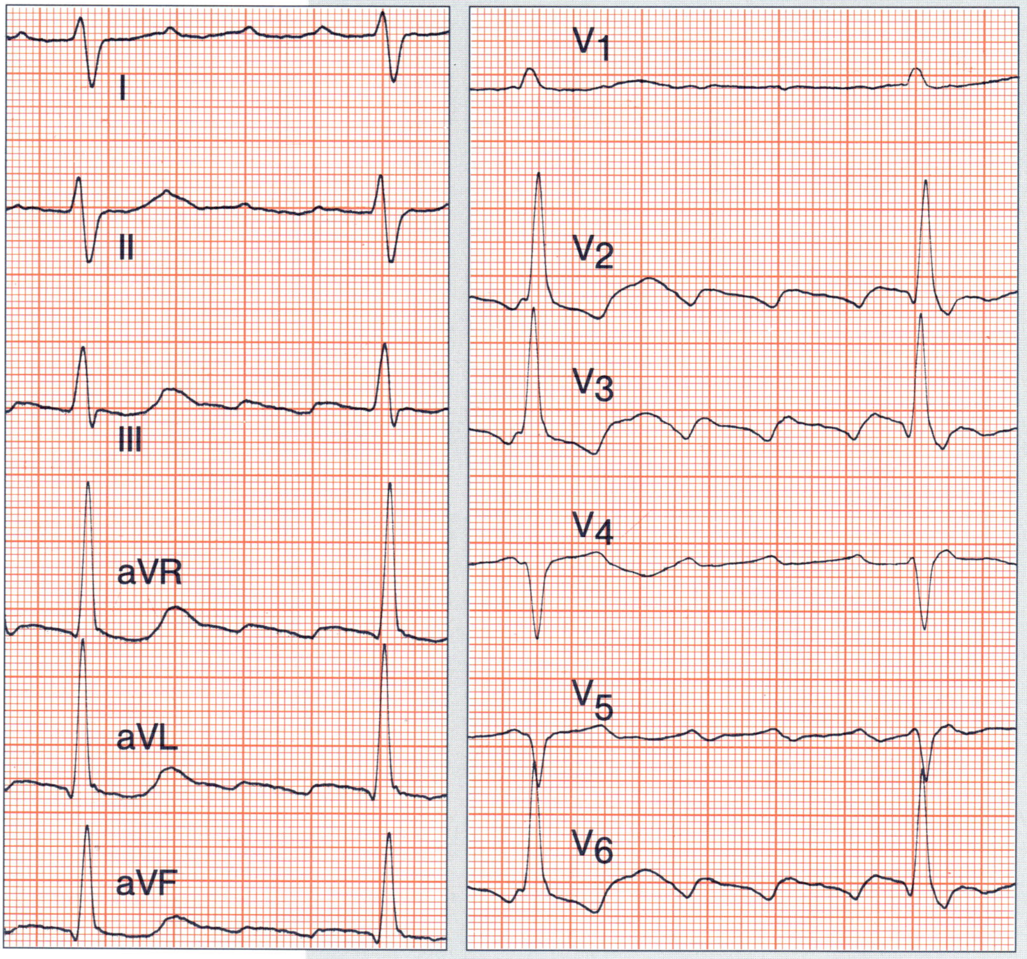

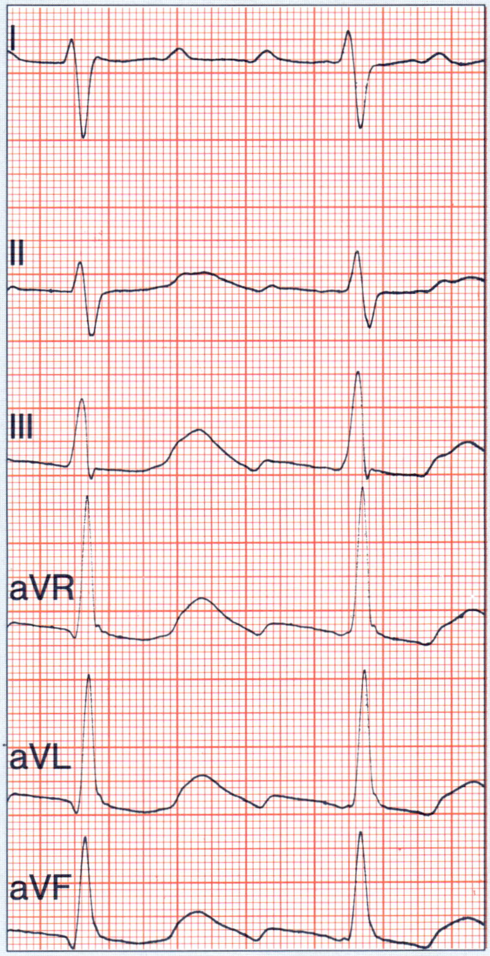
I
II
III
aVR
aVL
aVF

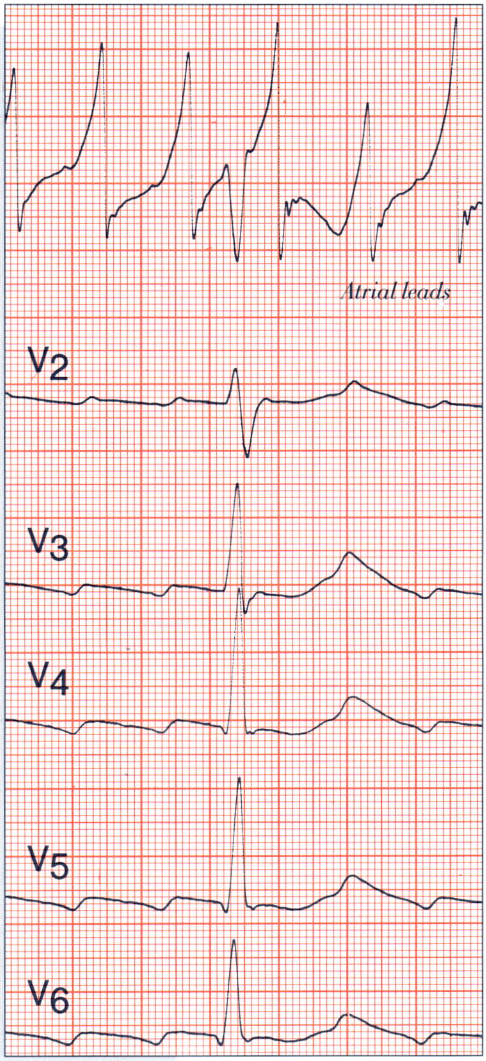
Atrial leads
V2
V3
V4
V5
V6

This ECG with 6 leads shows the burst during overstimulation and atrial fibrillation (page 103).

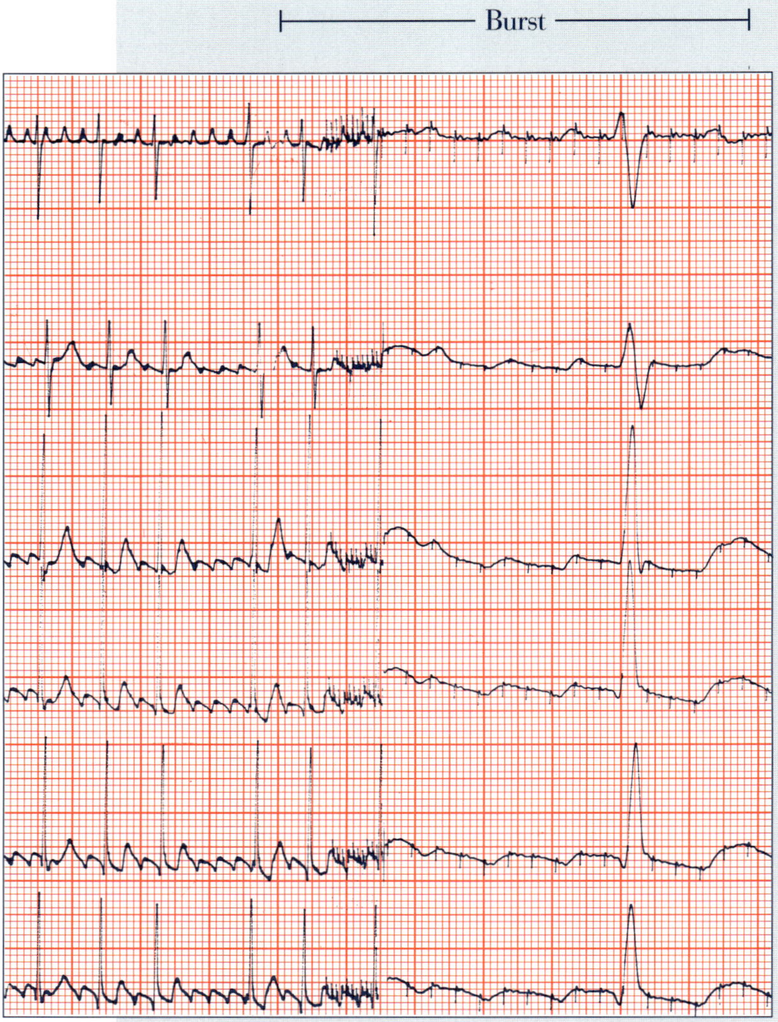

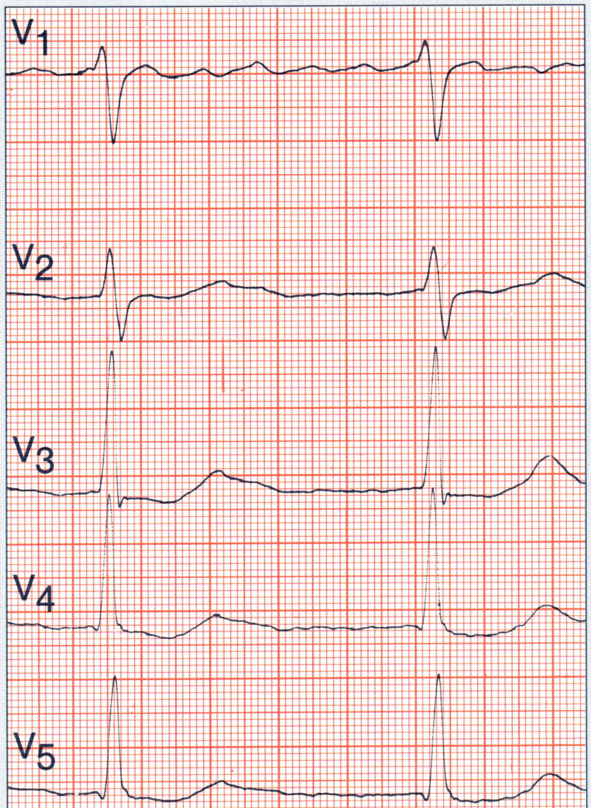
V1
V2
V3
V4
V5
V6

Same patient as before. Now there is a change to sinus rhythm and sinus bradycardia.

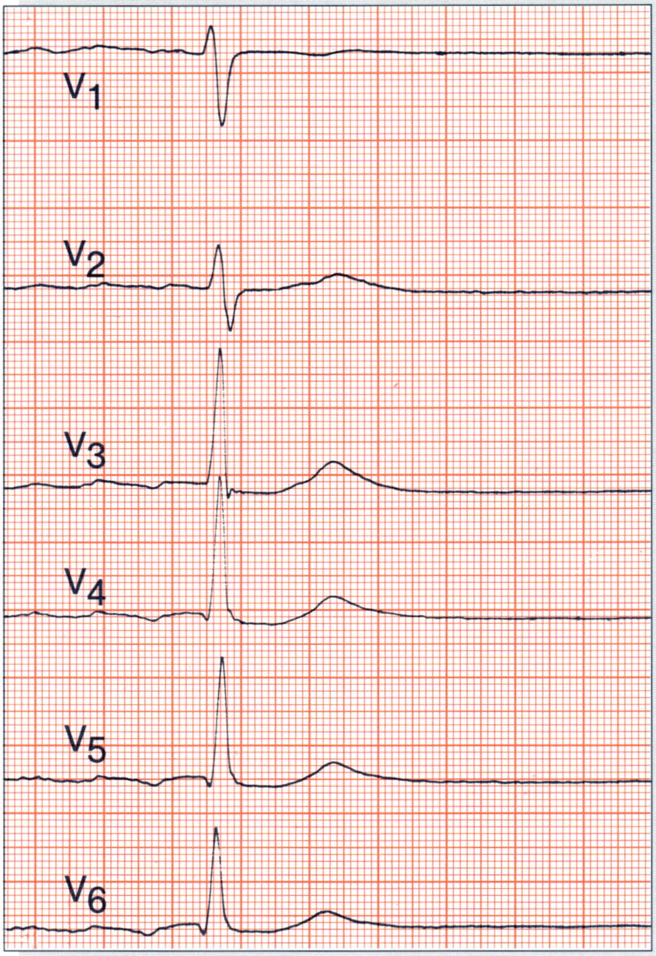

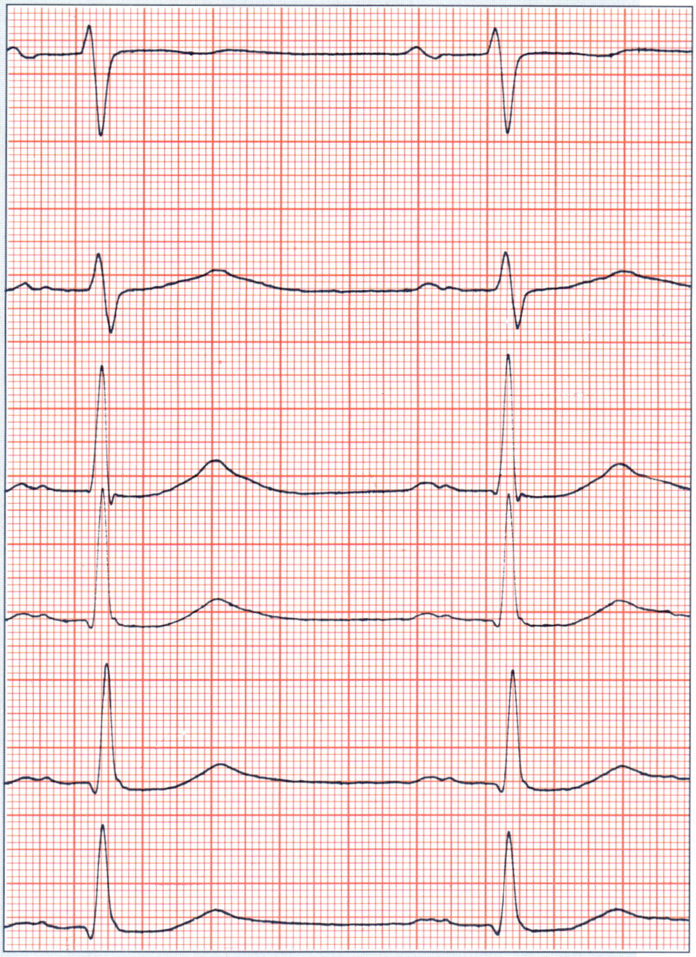

25-year-old sportsman with intermittent supraventricular tachycardias. During exercise testing there is a sudden increase in heart rate due to atrial tachycardia. The tachycardia was reversed into sinus rhythm with 25 mg ajmaline given intra-

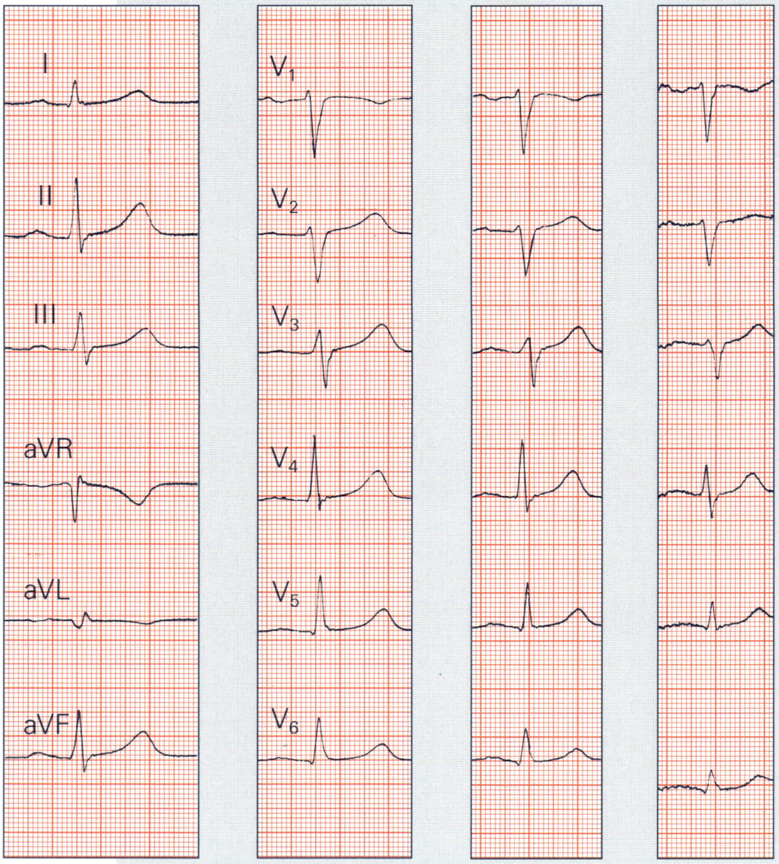

Rest *50 W* *100 W*

venously. The ECG at the top of the recording (this page) shows the advantage of continuous ECG recording during exercise testing, the arrhythmia is easily recognized and documented at the same time.

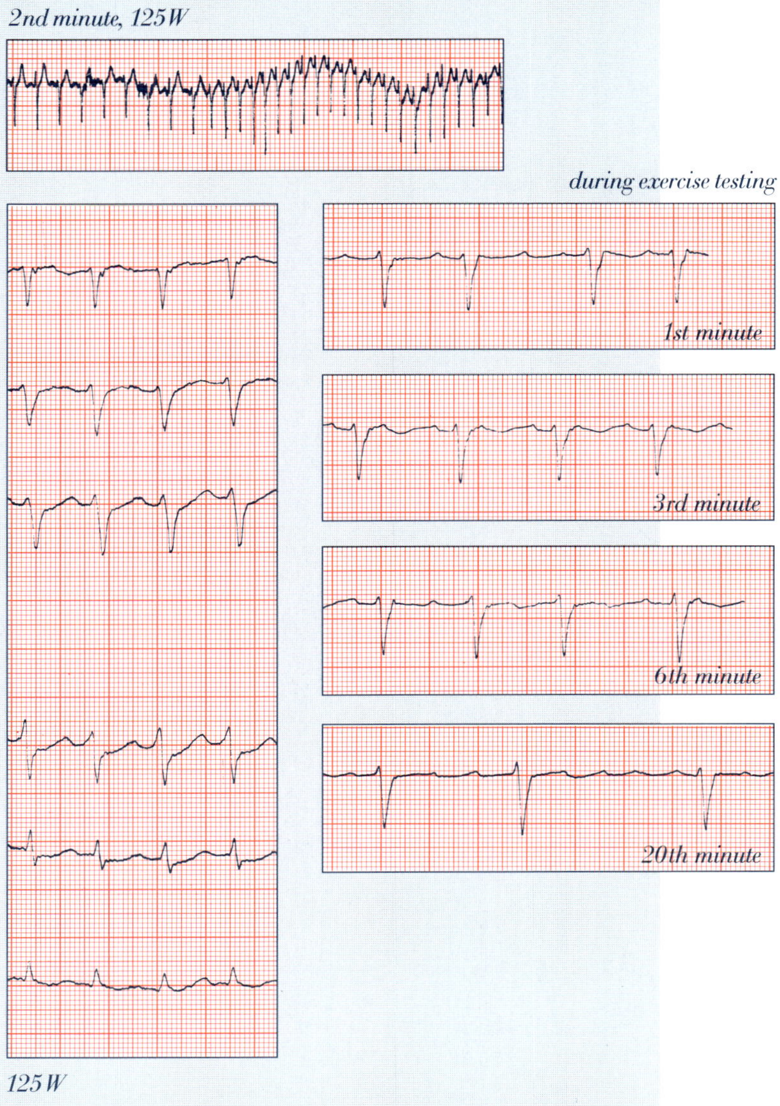

72-year-old patient with old myocardial infarction and paroxysmal supraventricular tachycardia with 2:1 conduction and wide QRS complex (a). This tachycardia yielded an un-

(a)

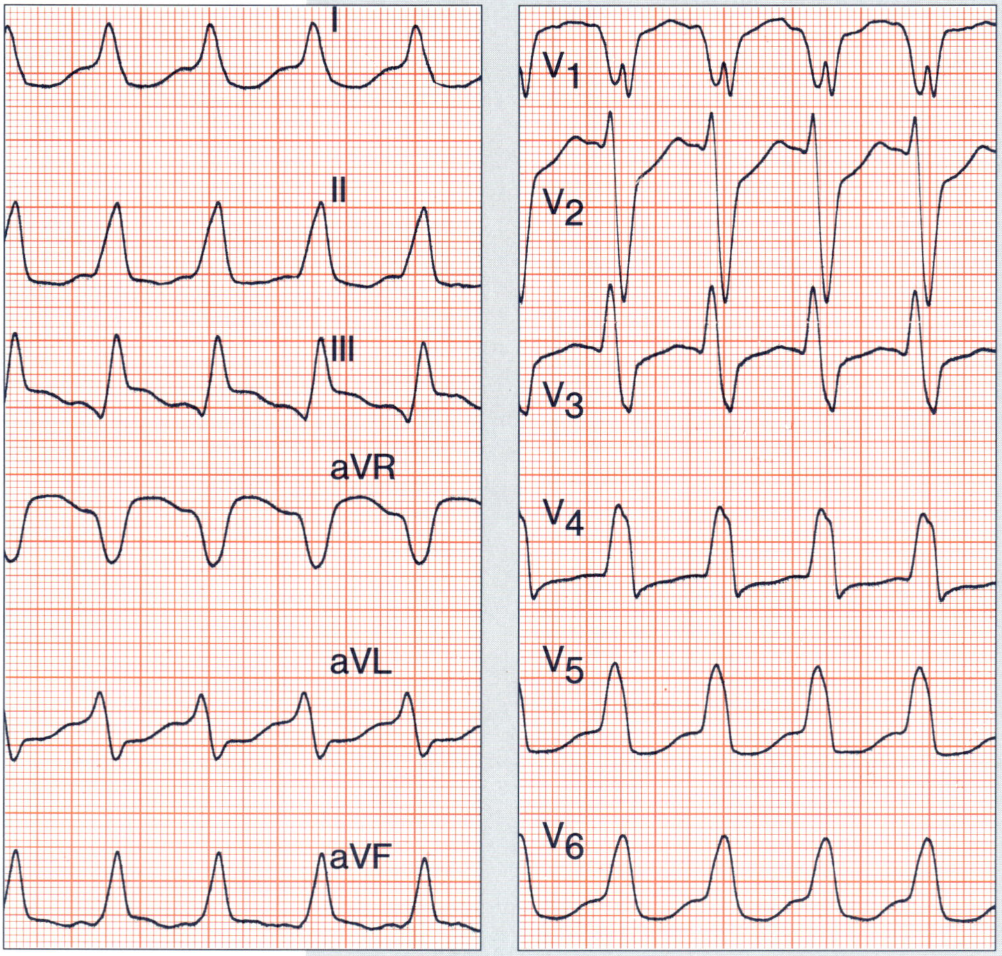

stable haemodynamic situation with drop in blood pressure. The patient underwent cardioversion with 25 J, followed by immediate sinus rhythm (b).

(b)

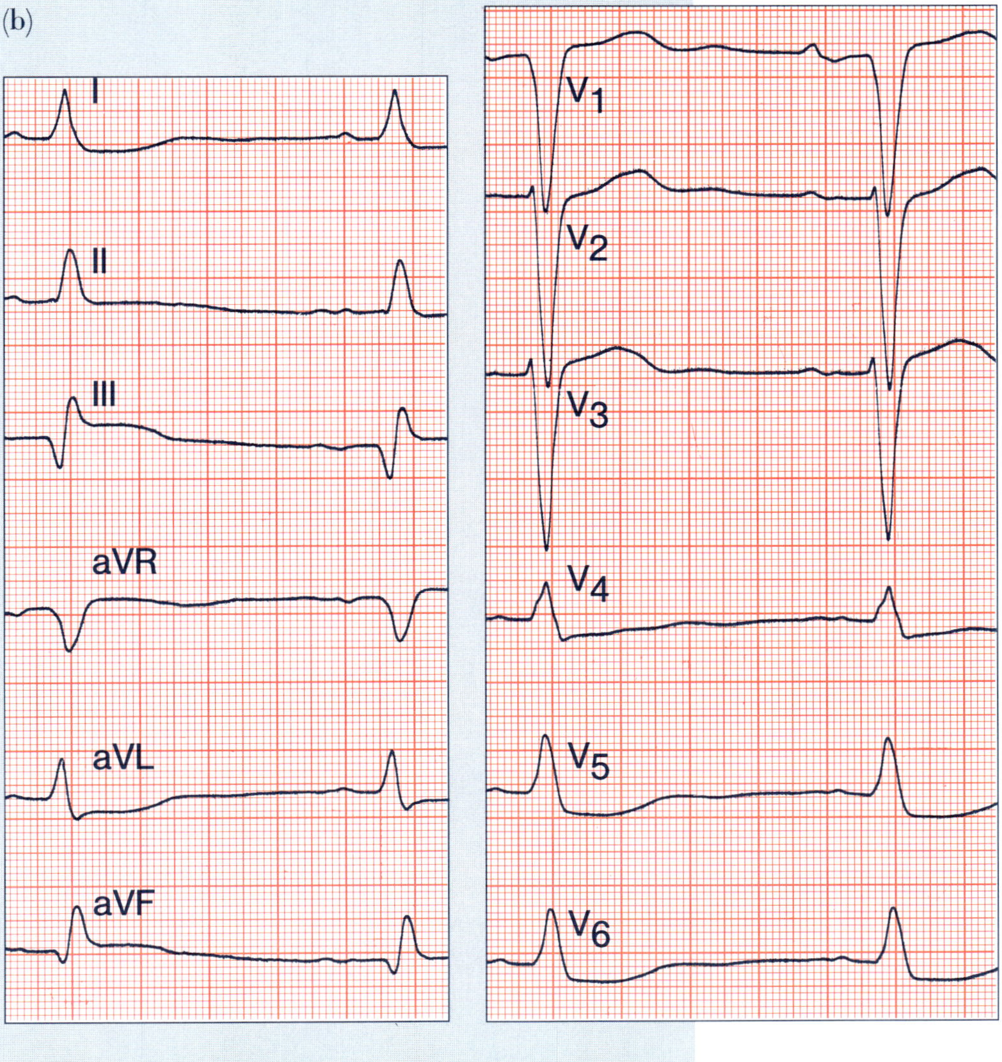

Supraventricular tachycardia showing the diagnostic significance of carotid pressure. During supraventricular tachycardia (left part of rhythm strip), pressure on the carotid shows

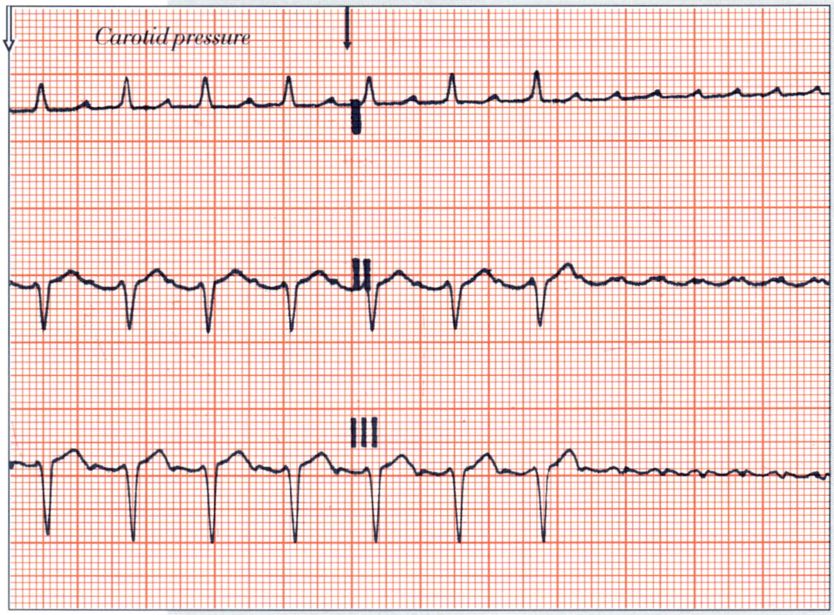

atrial flutter with very slow conduction. This vagal manoevre shows the diagnostic relevance in analysing supraventricular tachycardias.

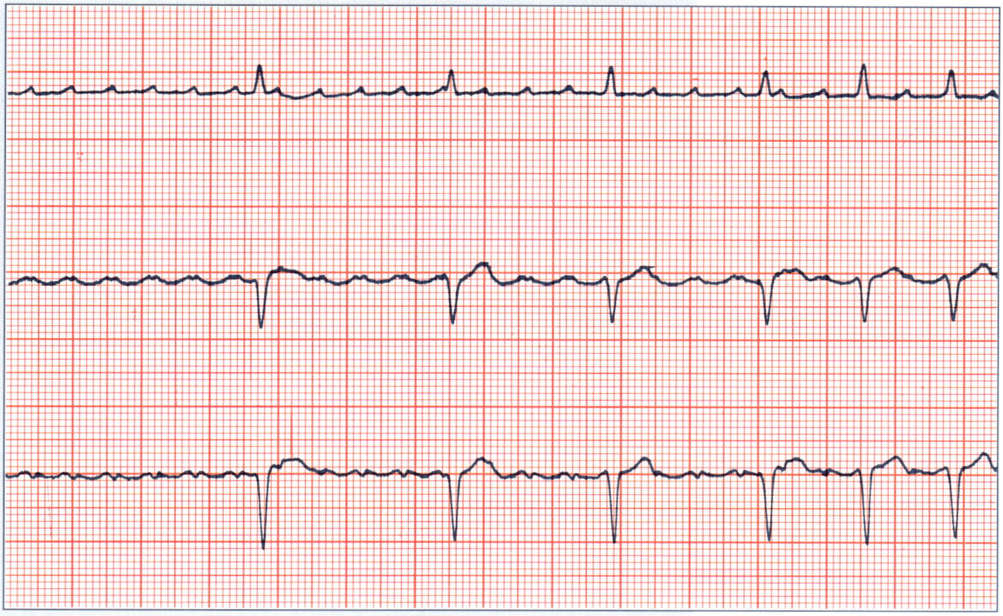

24-year-old female patient with ventricular arrhythmias without symptoms. The ECG was recorded during routine examination for sports activities. The ECG demonstrates ventricular parasystole with focal ventricular tachycardias. The diagnosis was confirmed by electrophysiological exami-

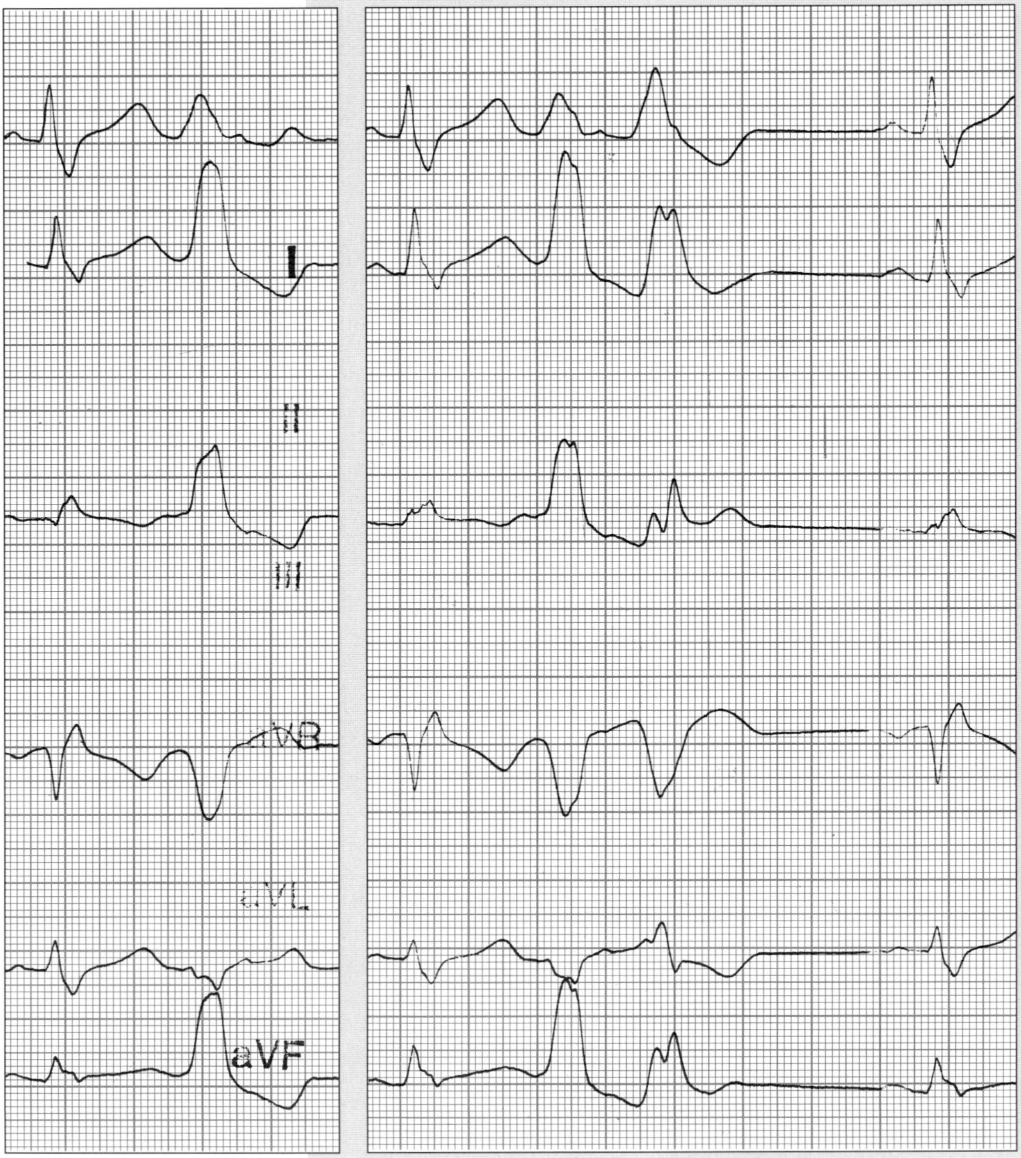

Rest

nation including ventricular stimulation. This kind of arrhythmia is benign in nature; in this case it disappeared after 2 years without any therapy. The exercise ECG shows salvos of ventricular extrasystoles.

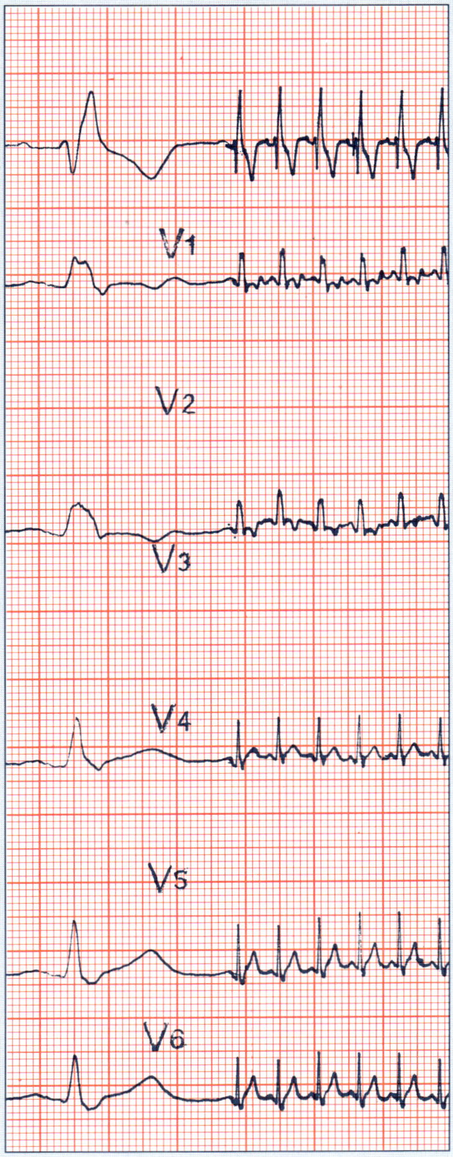

50W

Ambulatory recording of a 57-year-old patient with CAD and sudden cardiac death during ambulatory ECG. The first strip shows ventricular tachycardia (torsade de pointes), followed by ventricular flutter and ventricular fibrillation (b). Later on, there is electromechanical dissociation with some singular bradycardic extrasystoles (c).

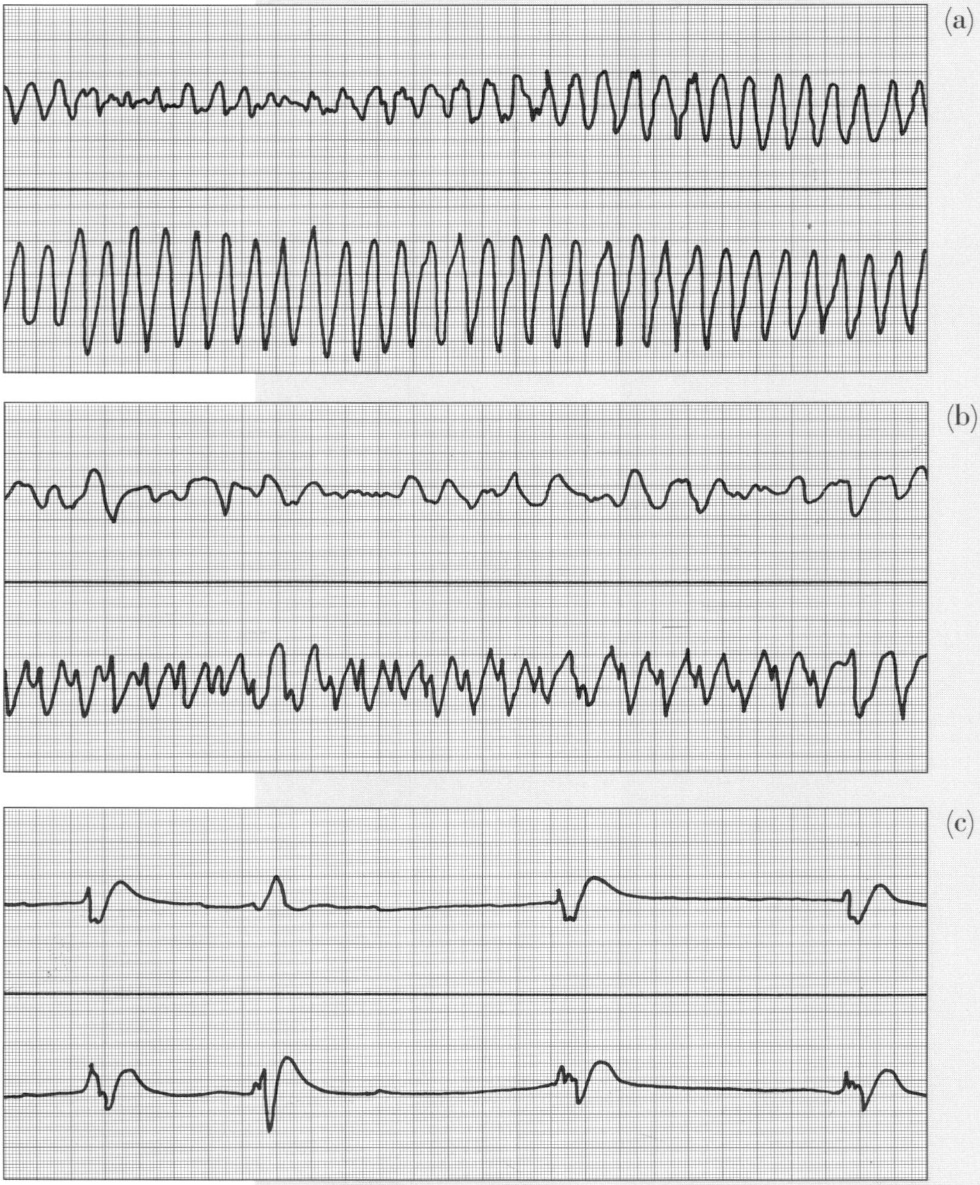

71-year-old patient with syncope after implantation of a pacemaker. The ambulatory ECG shows sustained ventricular tachycardia. In the right upper corner the reduced continuous recording is shown, and on the left, the 1:1 recording. The patient is suffering from dilated cardiomyopathy and was treated with amiodarone, which abolished all tachycardias.

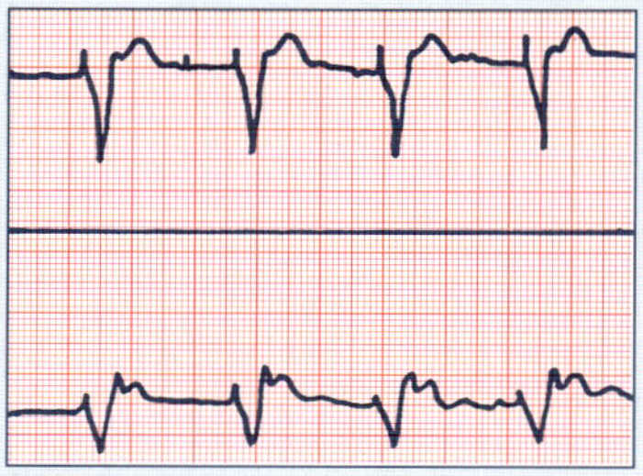

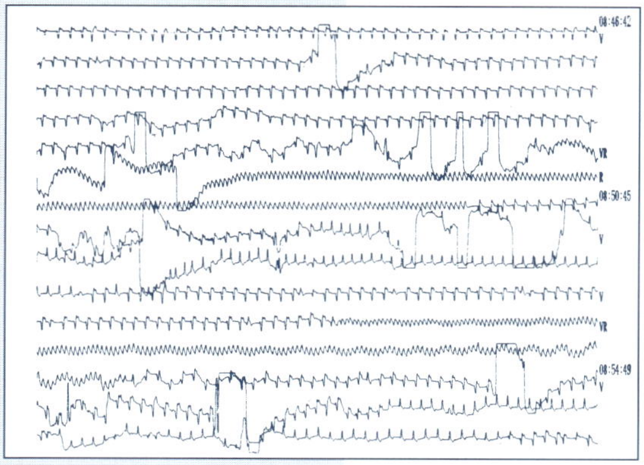

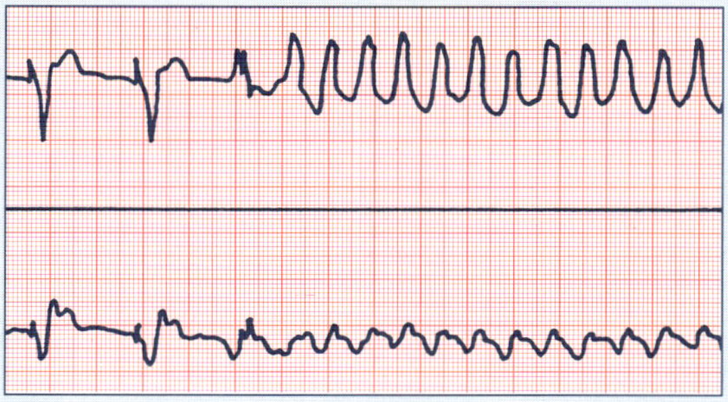

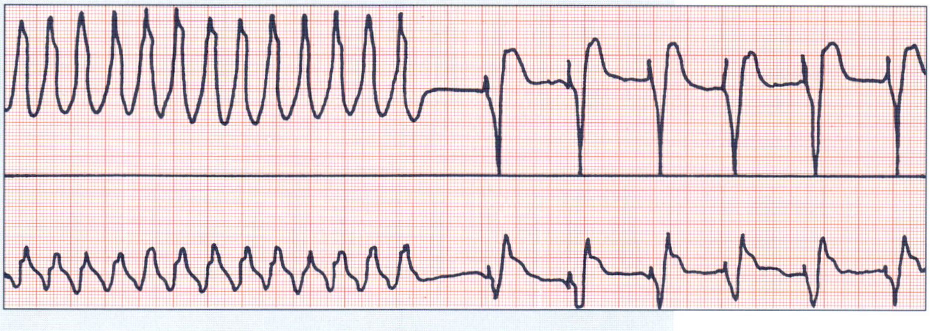

Resting and exercise ECG of a 19-year-old sportsman with syncope. At rest, repolarization abnormalities with negative T waves which were interpreted as changes due to endurance training. During exercise testing the T waves became positive. The ambulatory ECG (page 117) shows all kinds of ventricular arrhythmias with ventricular tachycardia, torsade

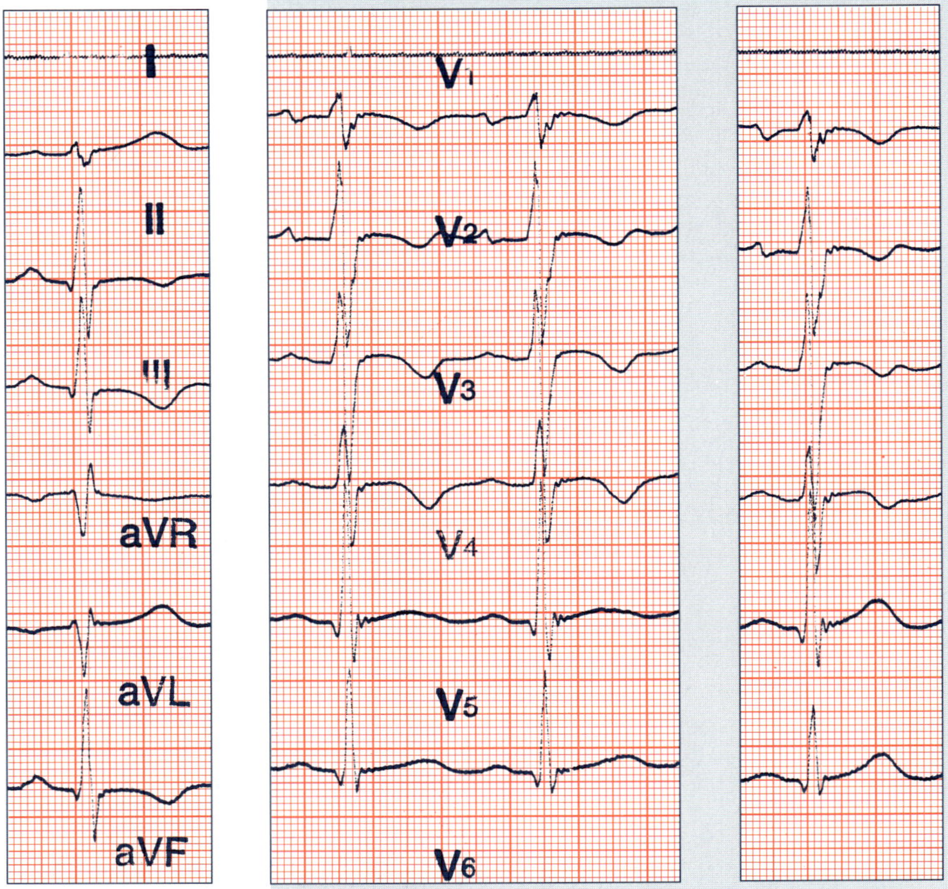

Rest

50W

de pointes, nonsustained ventricular tachycardia, ventricular extrasystoles and salvos. Myocardial biopsy revealed hypertrophic cardiomyopathy. The patient was treated with beta-blockers; this abolished all ventricular arrhythmias.

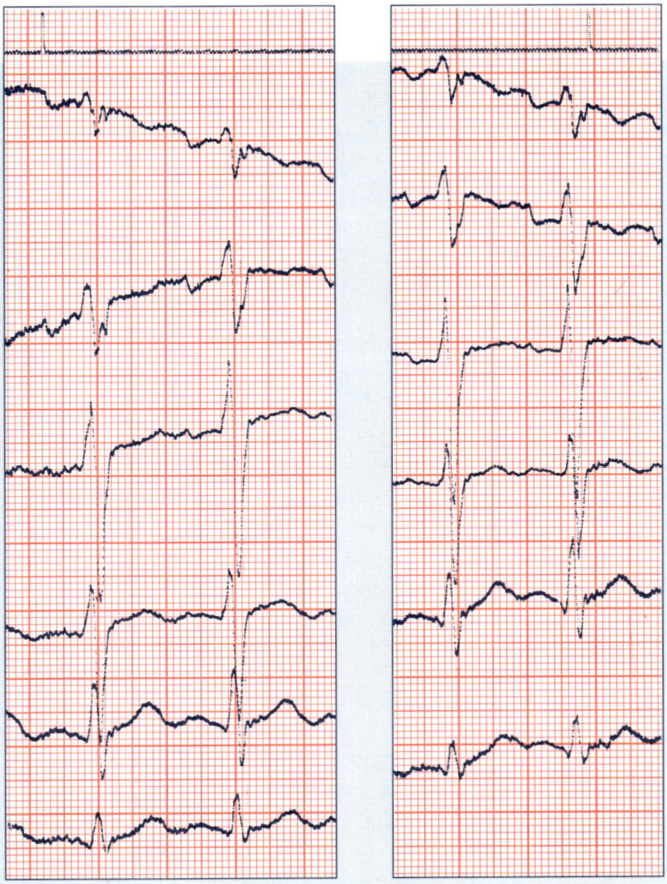

150 W *200 W*

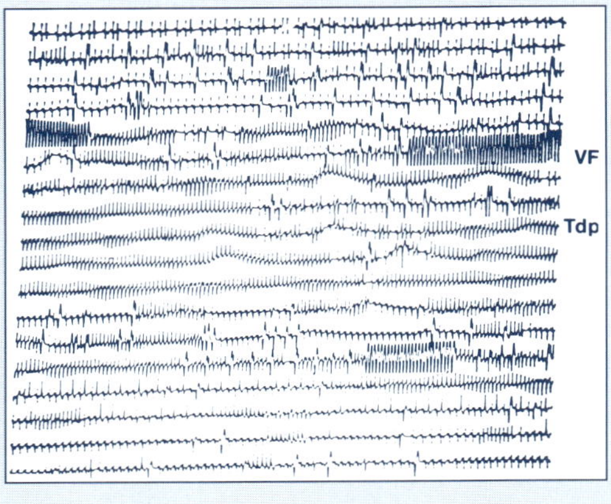

40-year-old patient without symptoms and good exercise tolerance. At rest, left bundle branch block (LBBB). The patient was examined to clarify the cause of LBBB. During exercise testing no symptoms occurred and the patient reached 150 W. Three minutes after end of exercise testing, there was

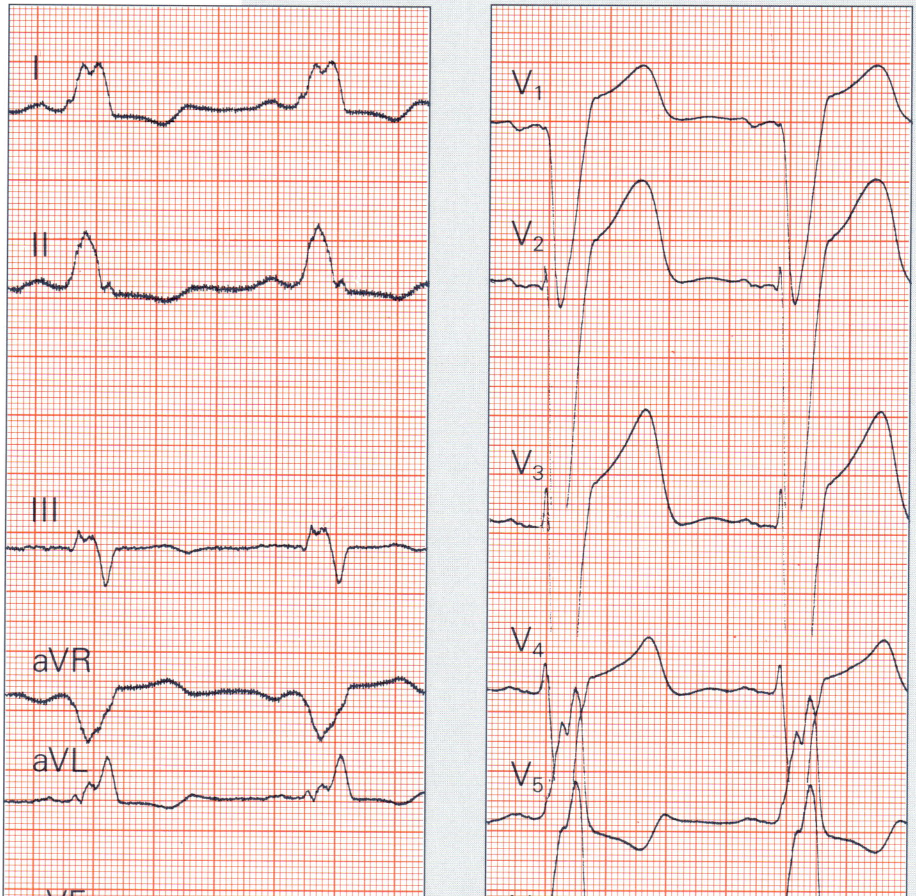

before exercise

sudden ventricular flutter. The patient was defibrillated with 200 J resulting in sinus rhythm. Right and left heart catheterization revealed an early stage of dilated cardiomyopathy.

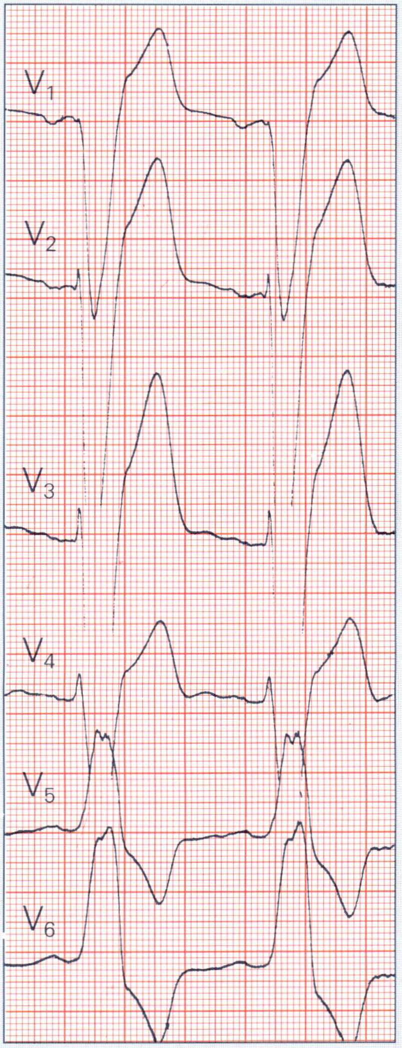

150 W max.

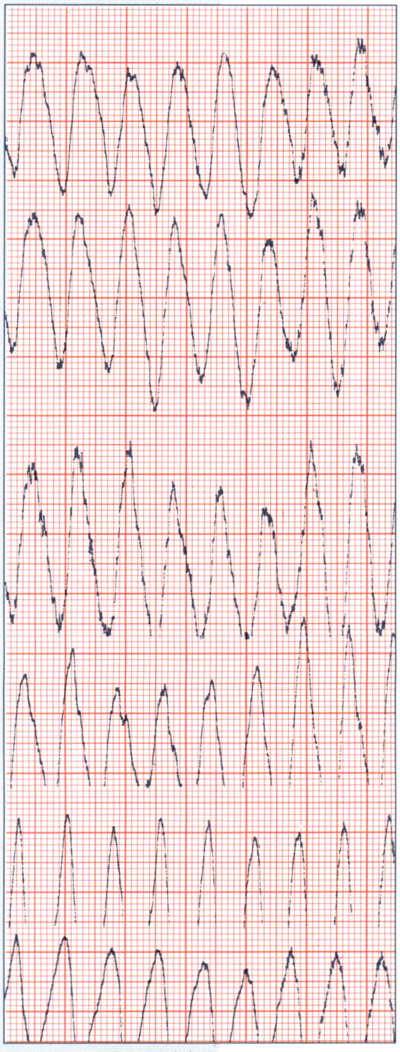

3 mins. rest after exercise

79-year-old patient with an old myocardial infarction and an intermittent rate-dependent LBBB.

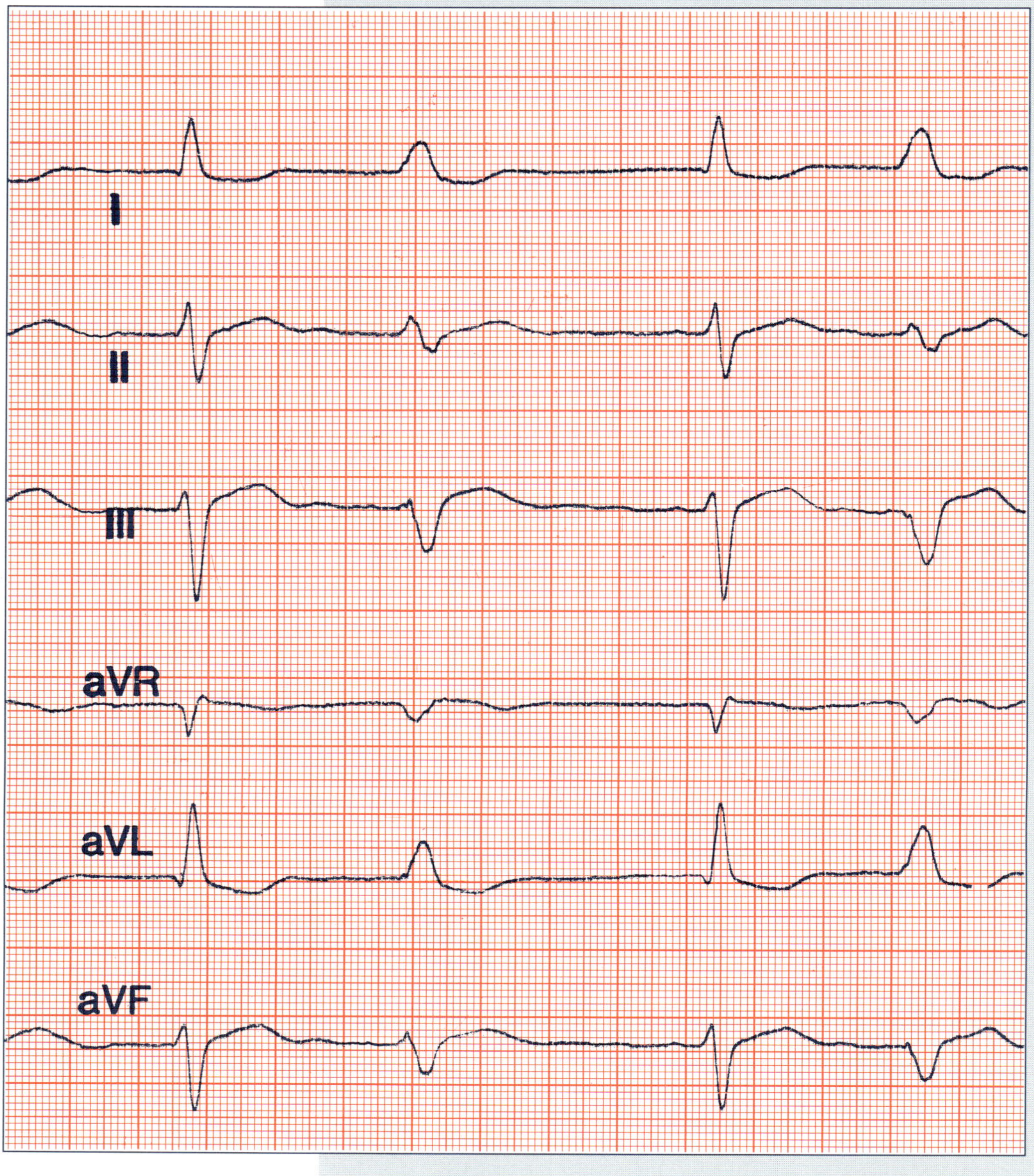

(Rhythm strip continued)

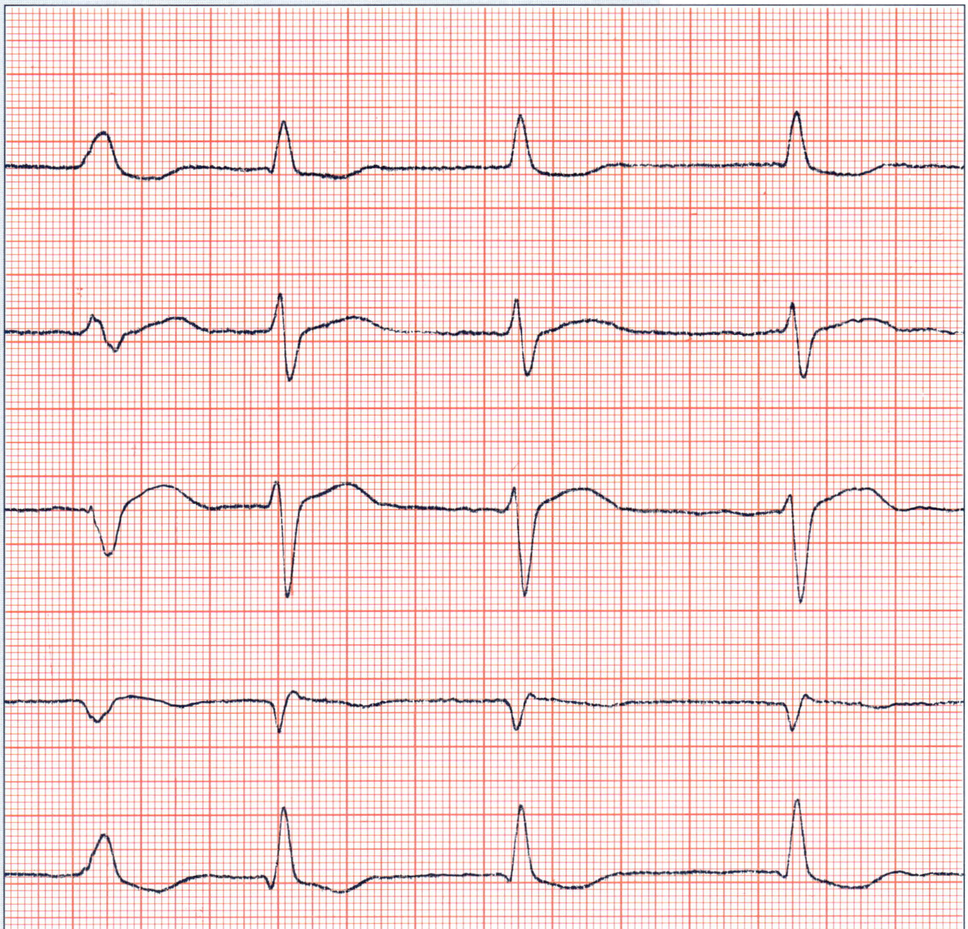

28-year-old patient, football player with syncope during a football game. He was resuscitated by an emergency physician who injected ajmaline and reversed ventricular fibrillation to atrial fibrillation. In the emergency ward there was atrial

(a)

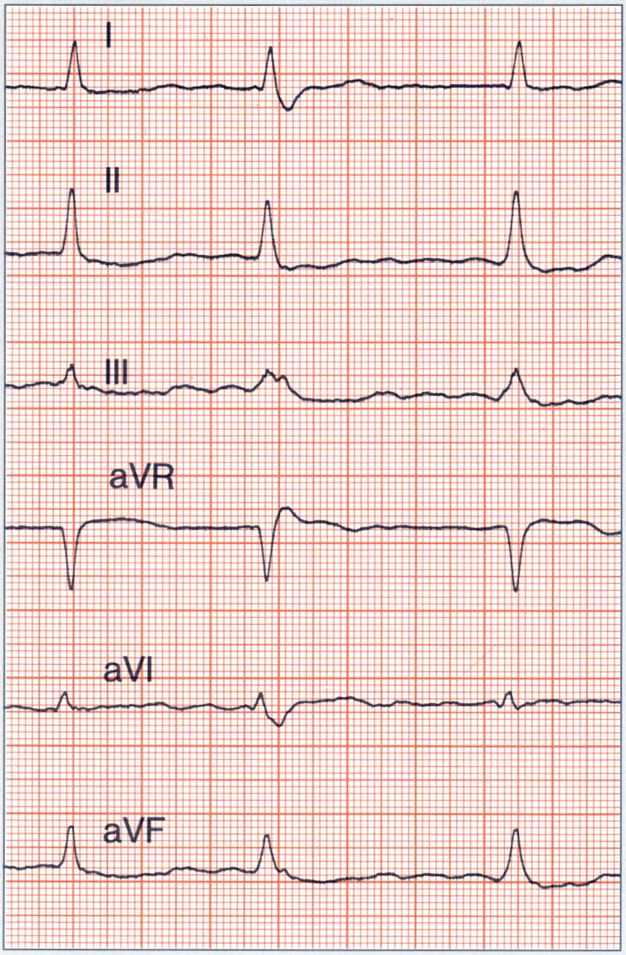

fibrillation (a) with sometimes rapid conduction, later on there was 1:1 conduction [page 124 (b)] and the patient again received ajmaline 50 mg i.v. This then converted the arrhythmia to sinus rhythm.

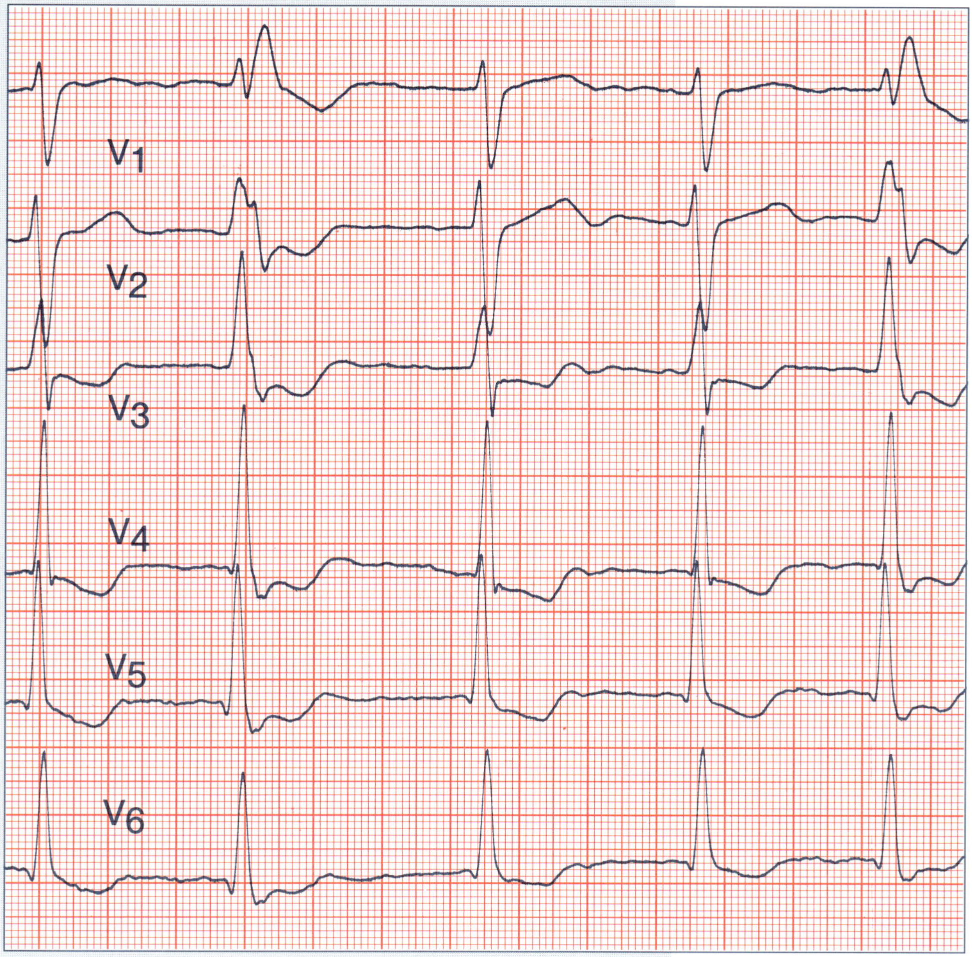

The same patient as before: this ECG shows preexcitation syndrome (WPW syndrome).

(b)

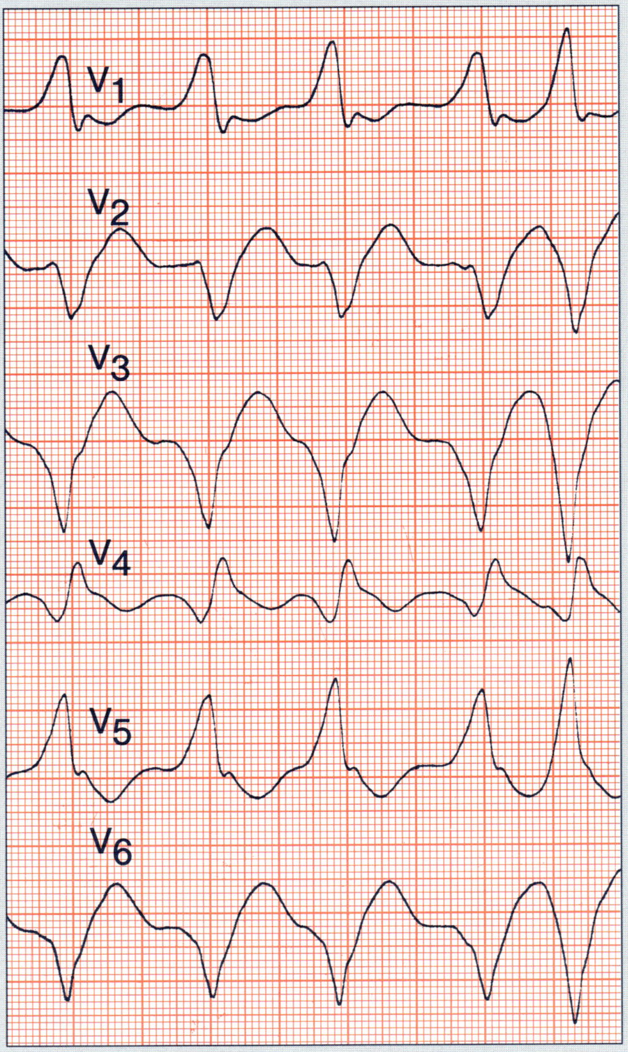

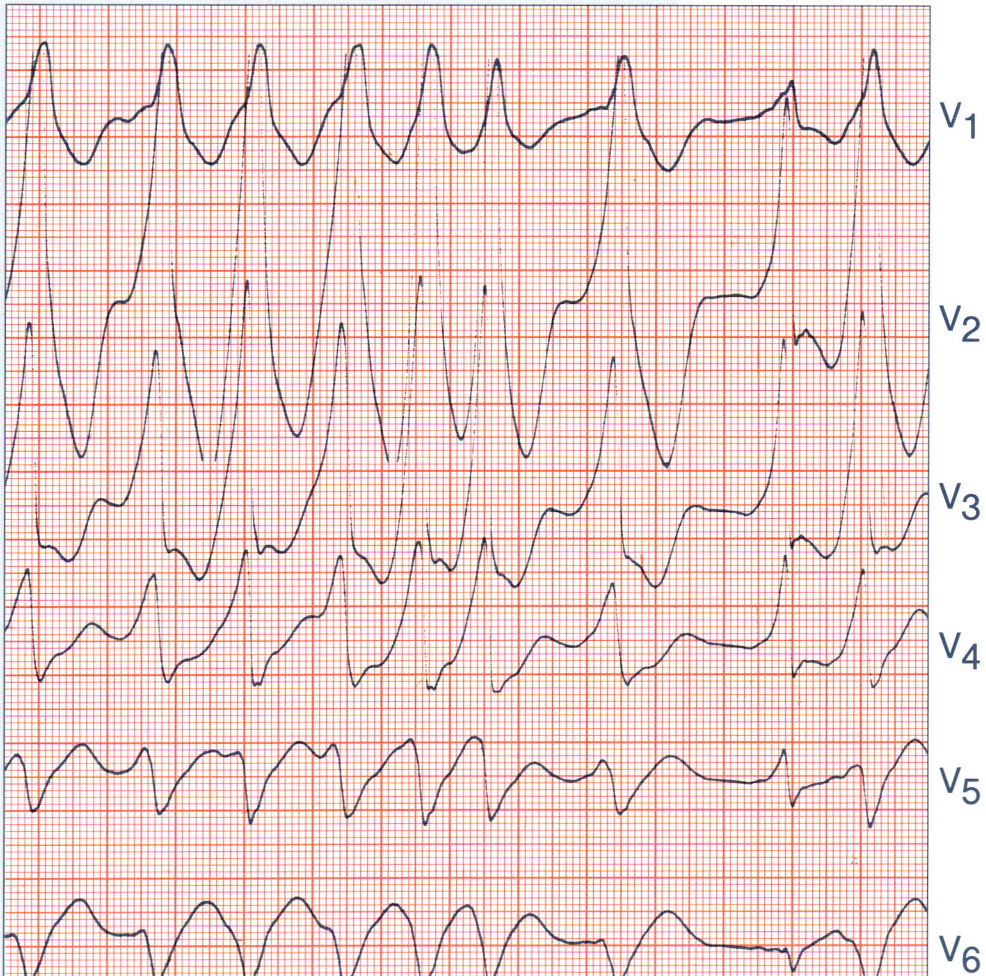

V1
V2
V3
V4
V5
V6

The same patient as on pages 124-125.

(c)

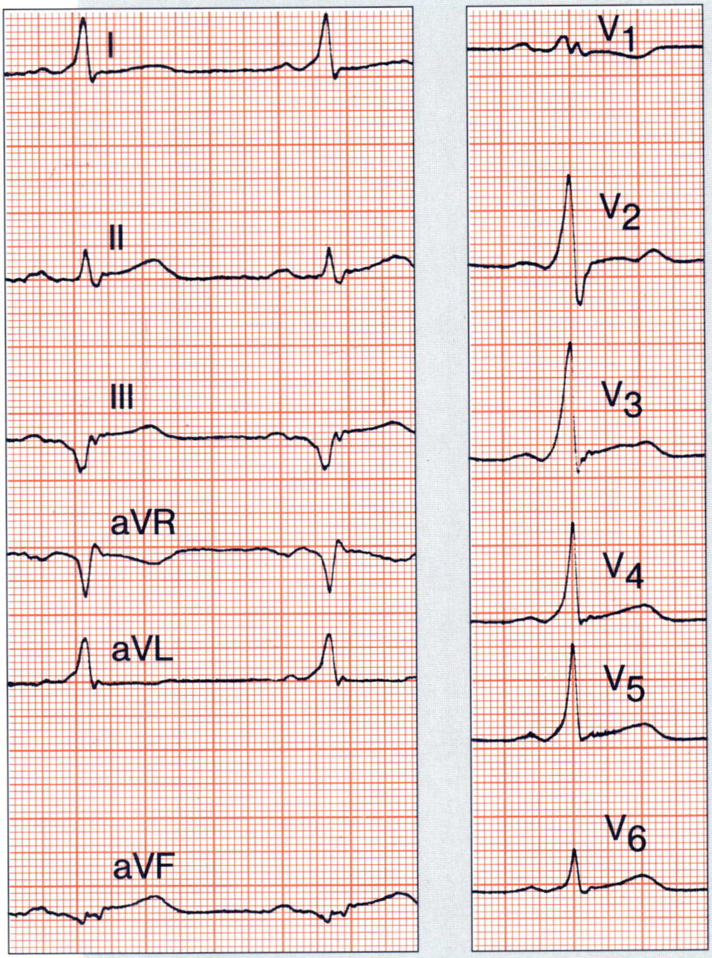

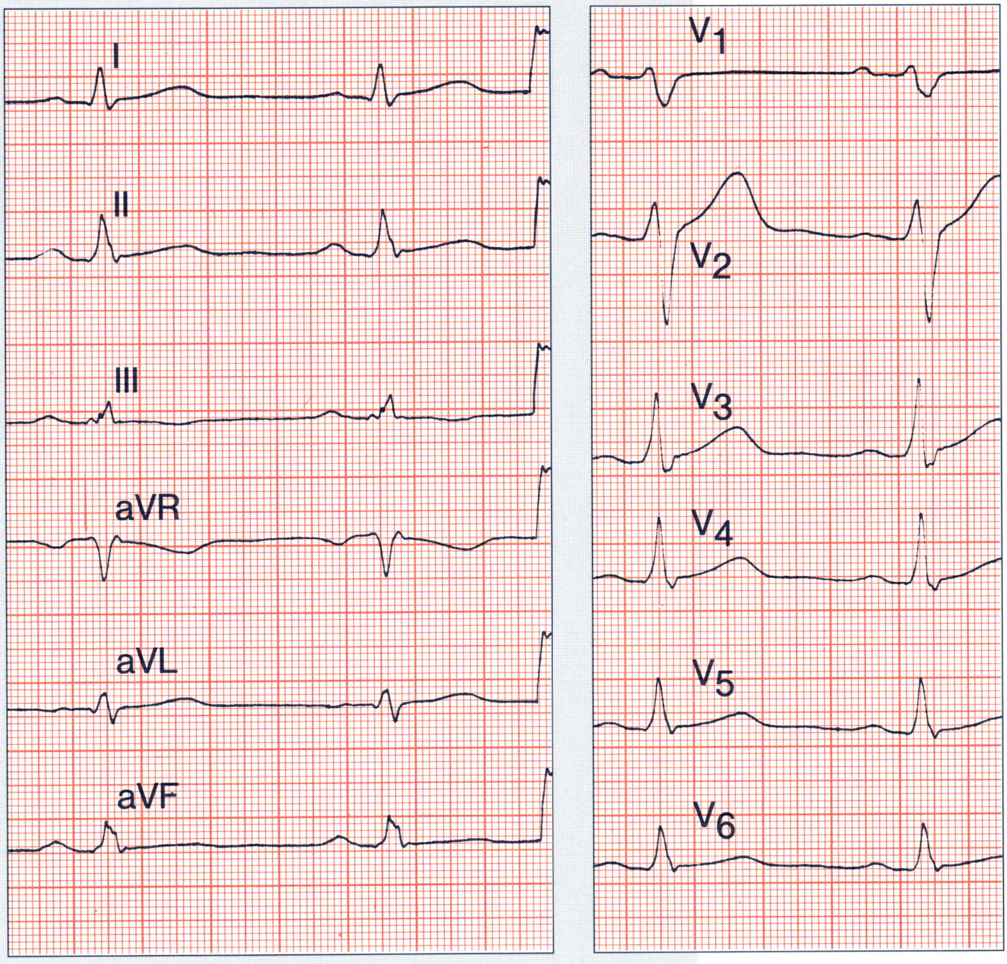
I
II
III
aVR
aVL
aVF
V1
V2
V3
V4
V5
V6

62-year-old patient with atrial fibrillation. The underlying heart disease was hypertension and CHD. Arrows indicate so-called aberration with a right bundle branch block configuration.

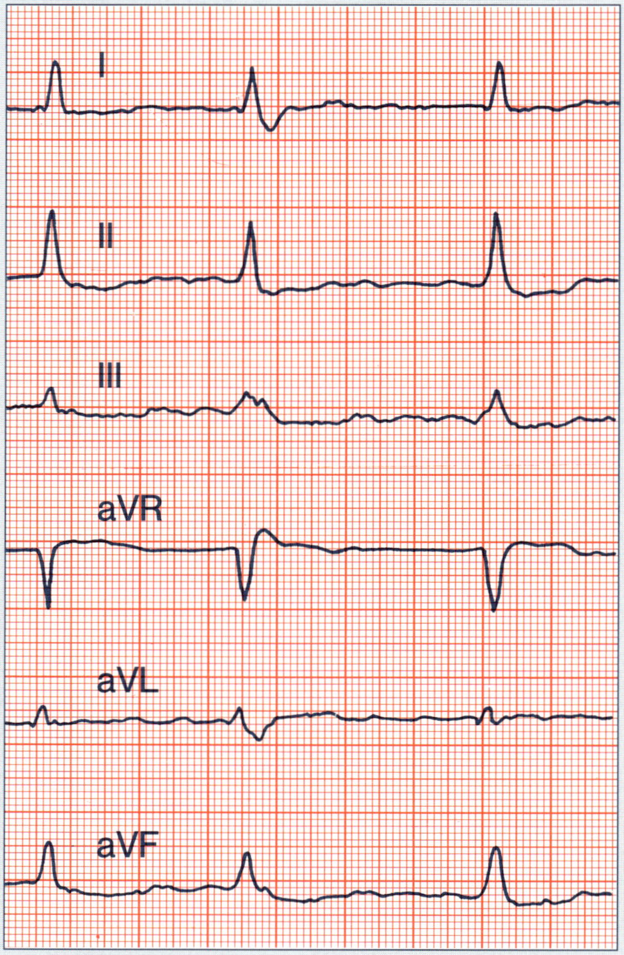

In addition, this ECG shows left hypertrophy and repolarization abnormalities due to left heart hypertrophy. These changes cannot be interpreted as being due to CAD or ischaemia.

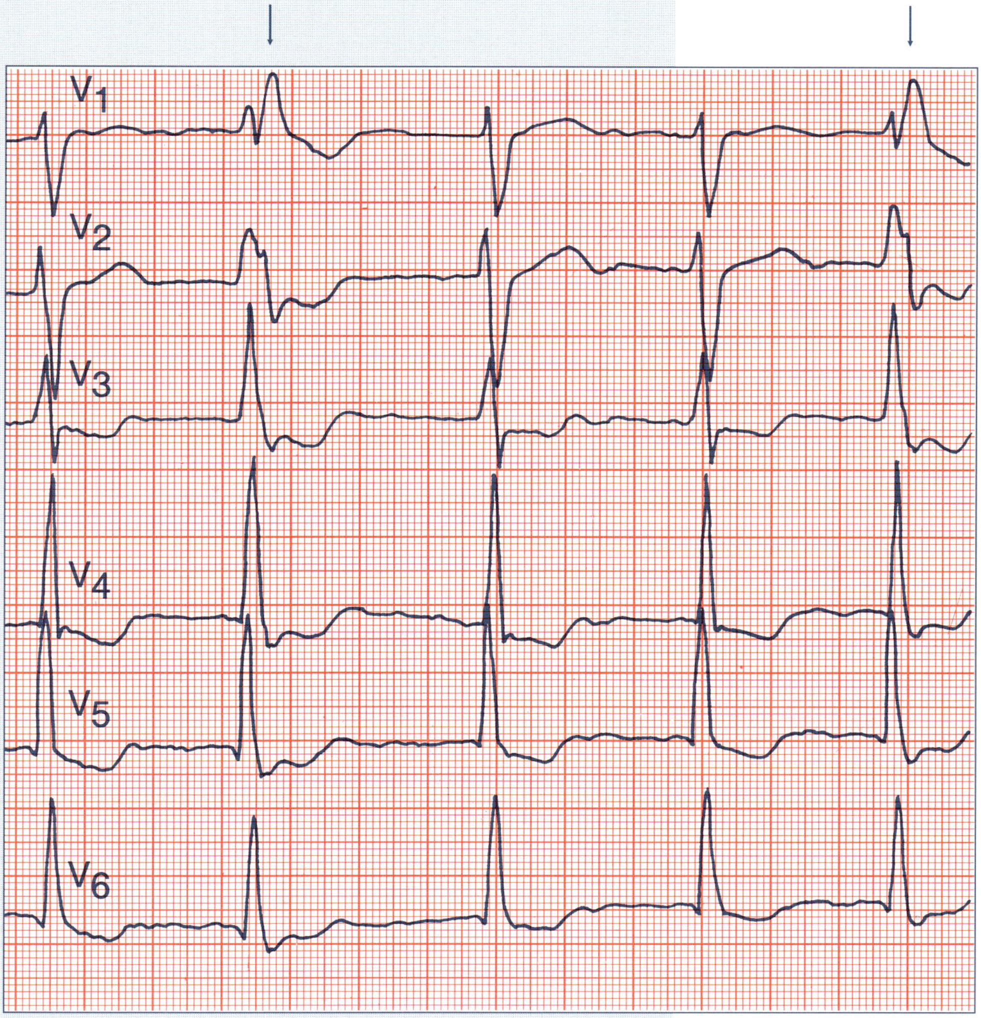

ECG showing tachycardia with wide QRS complex. The oesophagus lead (Ö) shows atrial (A) and ventricular (V) potentials which are independent of each other: Ventricular tachycardia due to CAD.

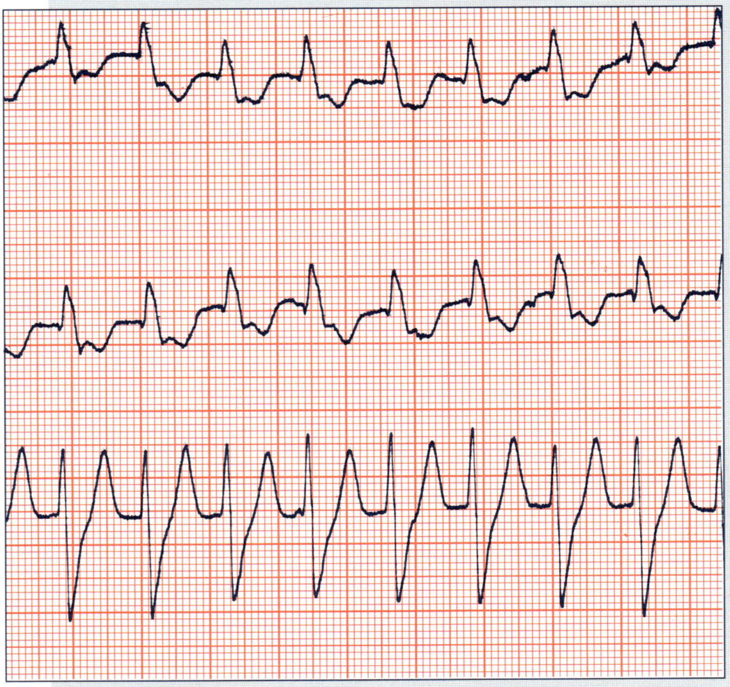

(Rhythm strip continued)

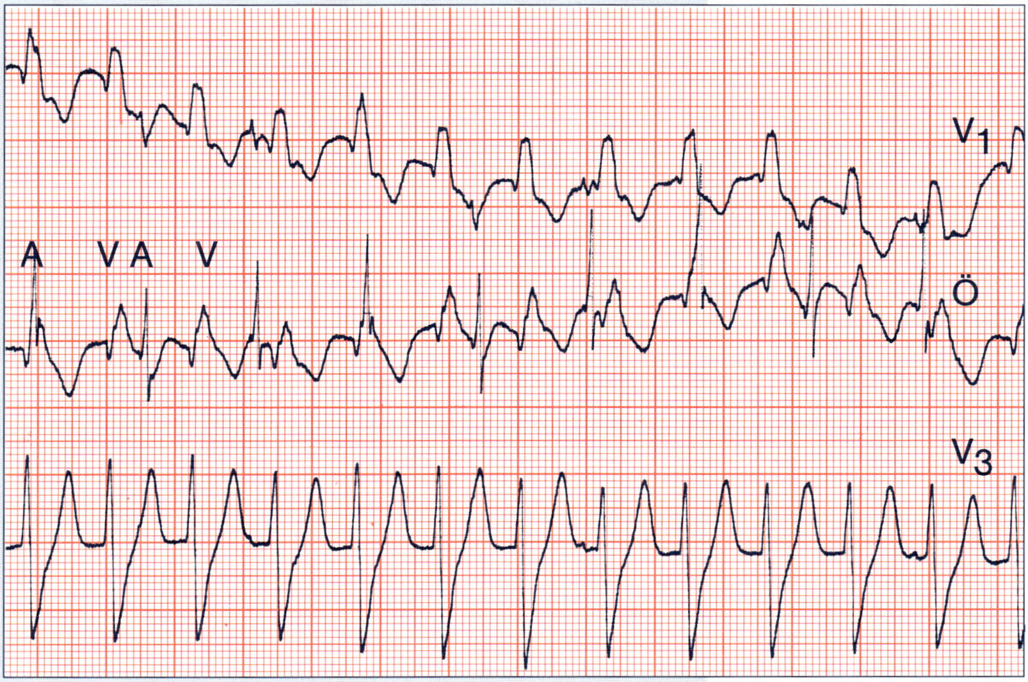

50-year-old female patient with CAD and severe 3-vessel disease. There is pronounced ST segment depression as a typical example of exercise-induced ischaemia. This recording

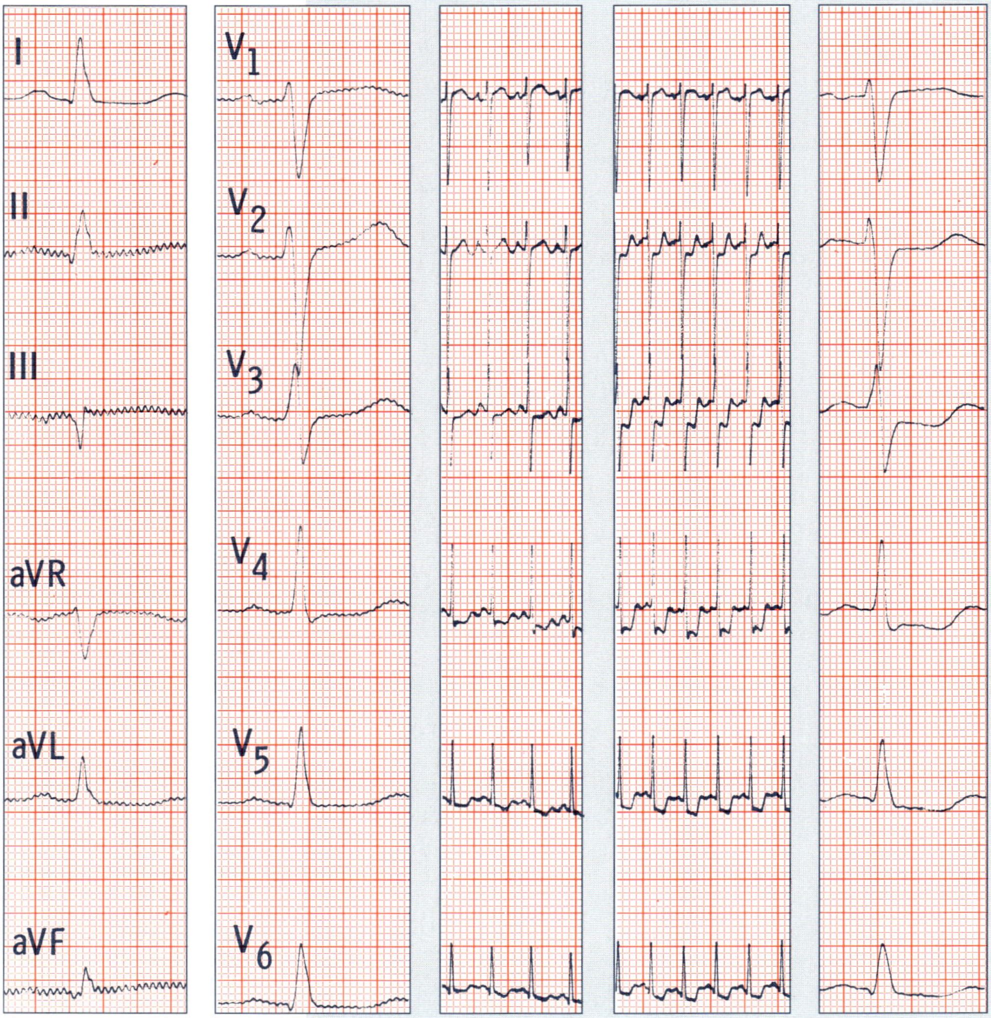

Rest

1st min.
25 W

2nd min.

also shows the advantage of continuous recording of the ECG during exercise testing at a low paper speed. Changes in the ECG can be easily recognized and are, at the same time, well documented.

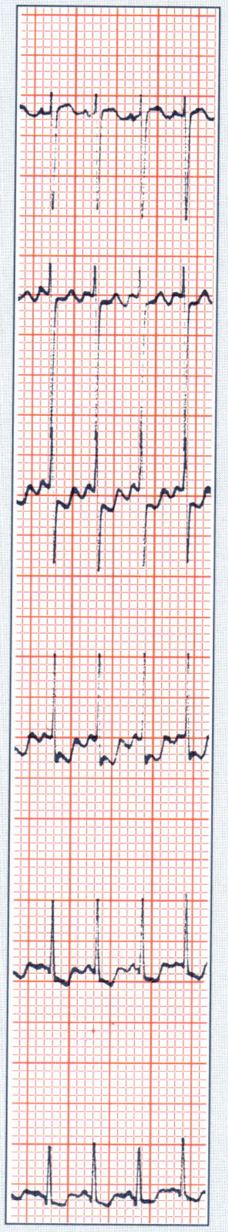

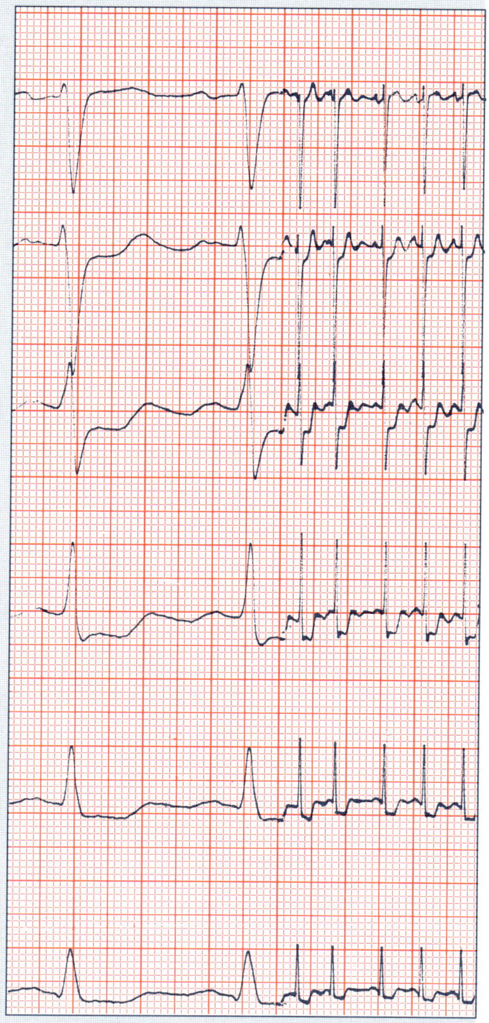

3rd min.
25 W

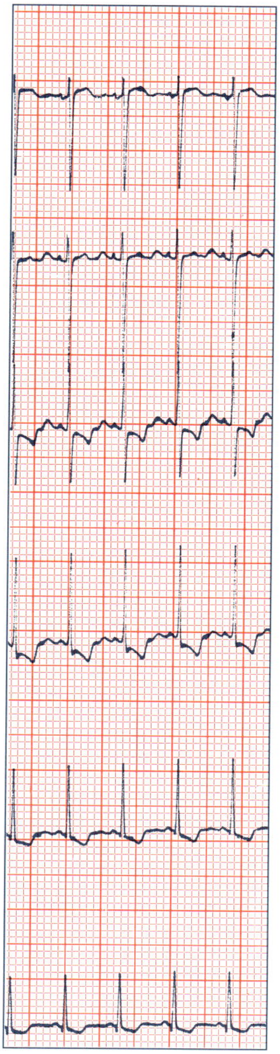

4 min. after exercise

44-year-old patient with severe stenosis of the R. interventricularis anterior (left anterior descending artery, LAD). Pronounced ST depression during exercise testing in combination with some extrasystoles.

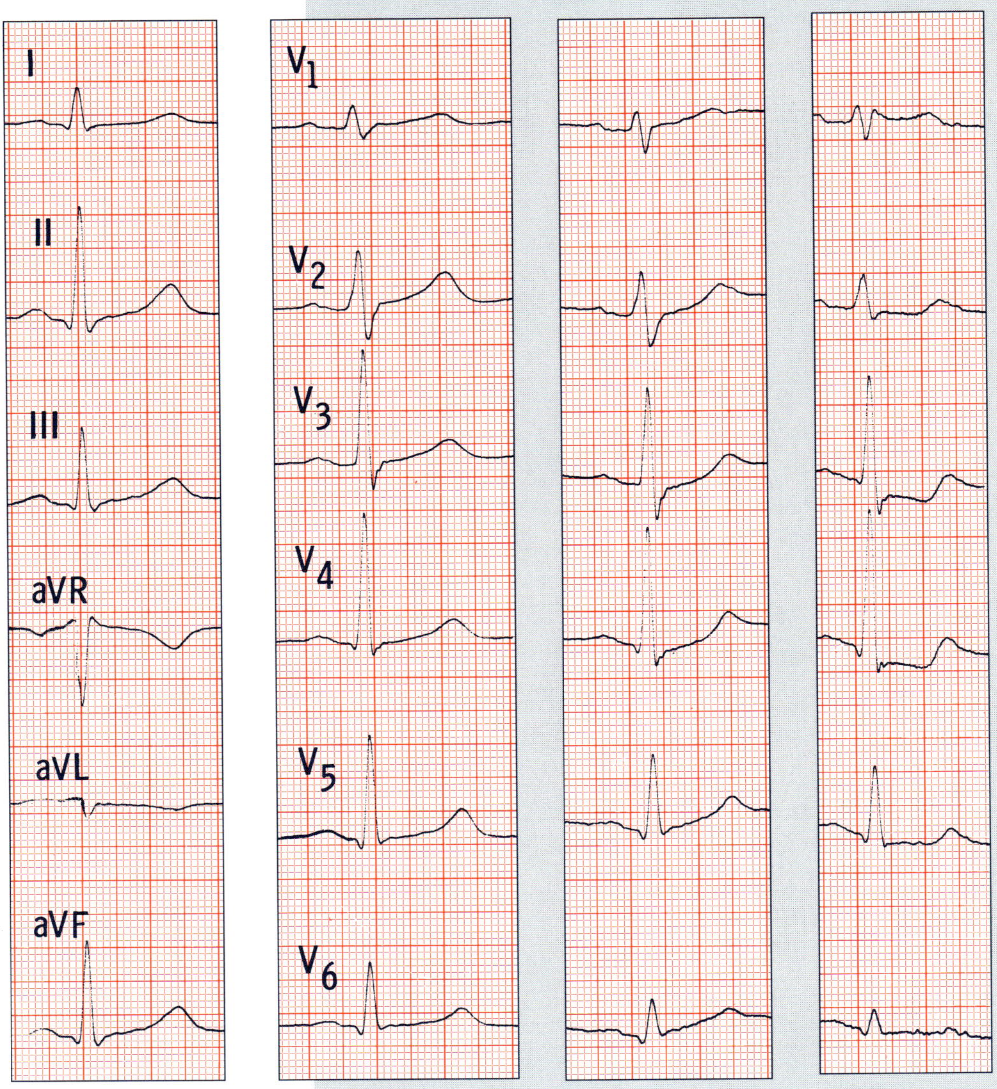

Rest *50W* *2nd min.*

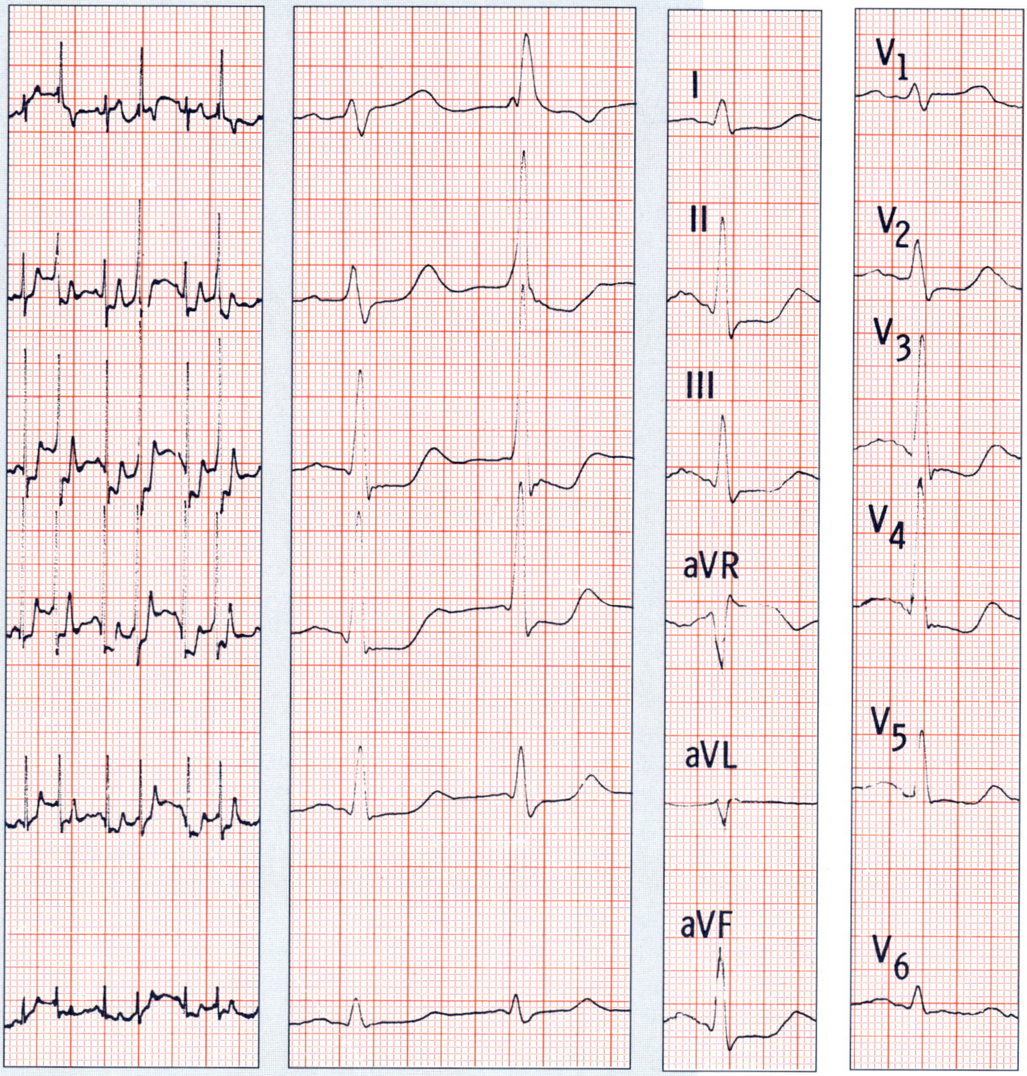

3rd min.
50 W

1st min.
75 W

immediately after exercise

The same patient as on page 134-135 after successful PTCA of the stenosis of the LAD. This example shows how interventions (treatment of coronary artery stenosis) can be documented by exercise testing.

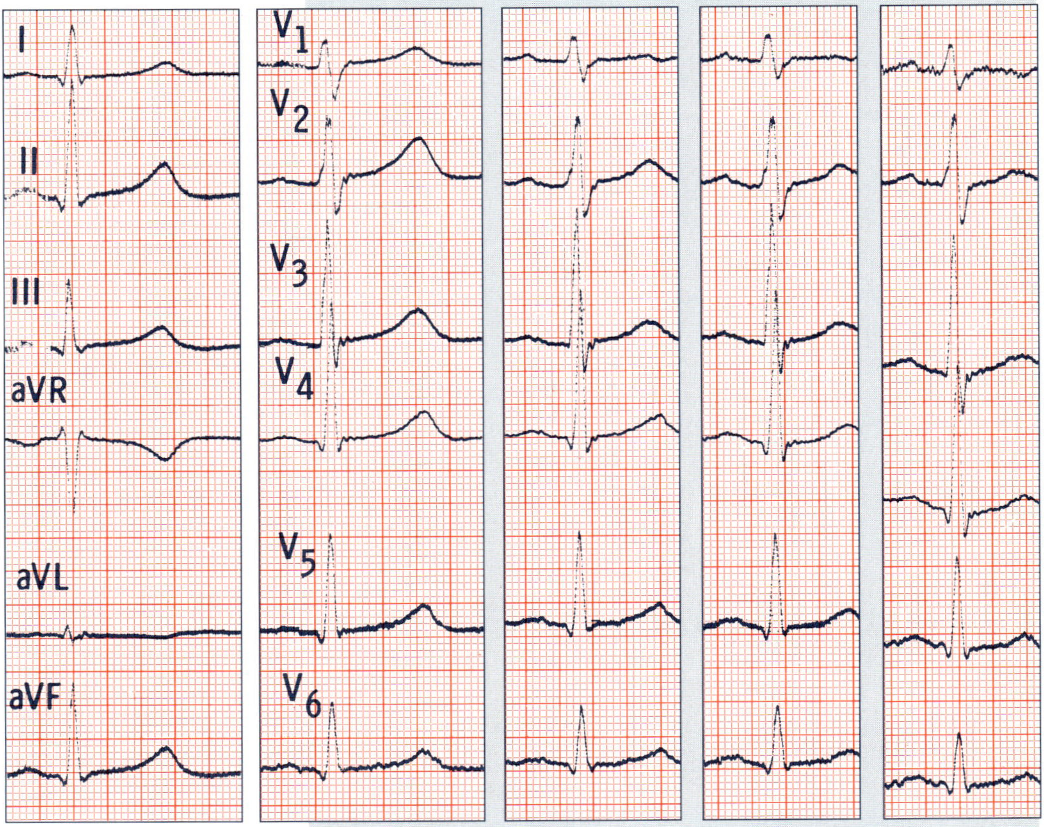

Rest *50W* *75W* *100W*

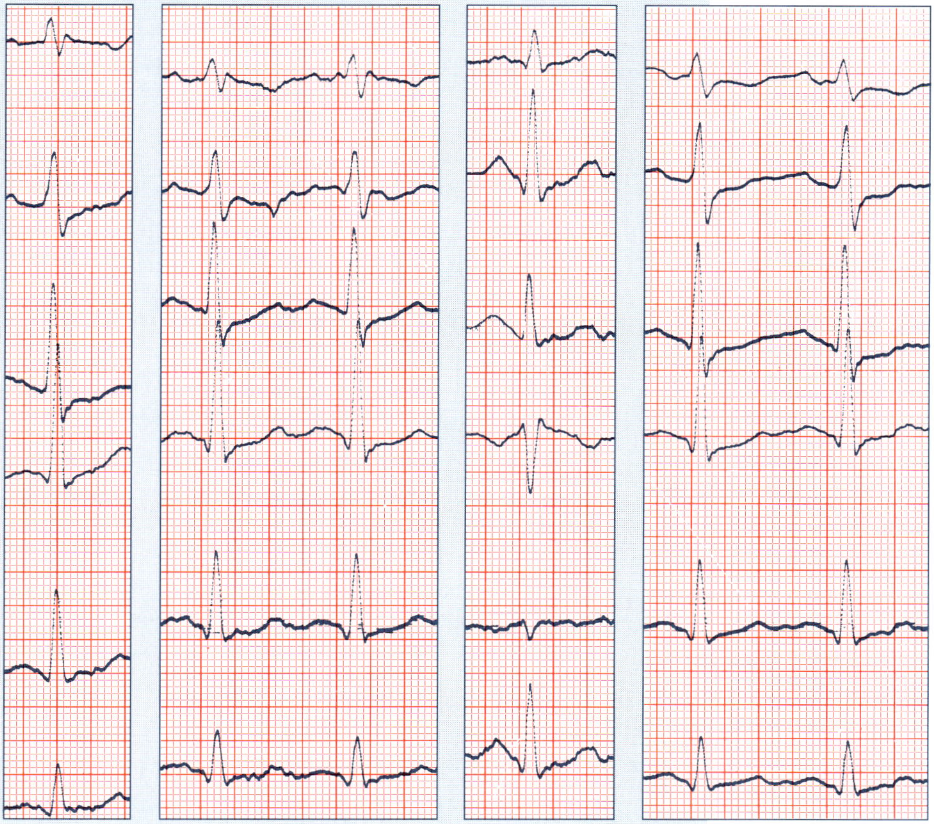

125 W *150 W* *immediately after exercise*

Ventricular arrhythmia due to dilated cardiomyopathy with paired ventricular extrasystoles. This is a pathological finding.

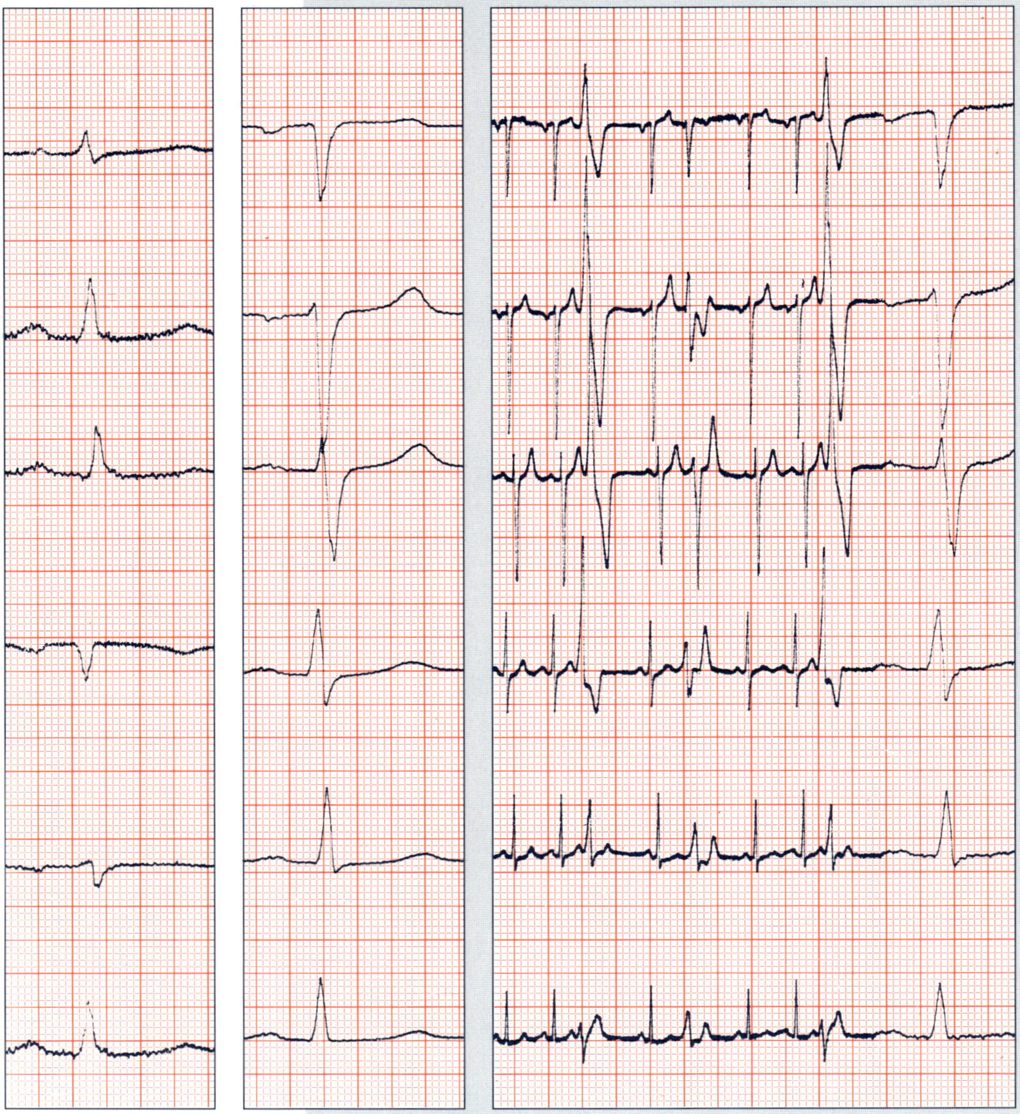

Rest *50W*

Consider: Exercise-induced ventricular arrhythmias may be due to cardiomyopathy or silent valve disease and cannot be assumed to be due to ischaemia alone.

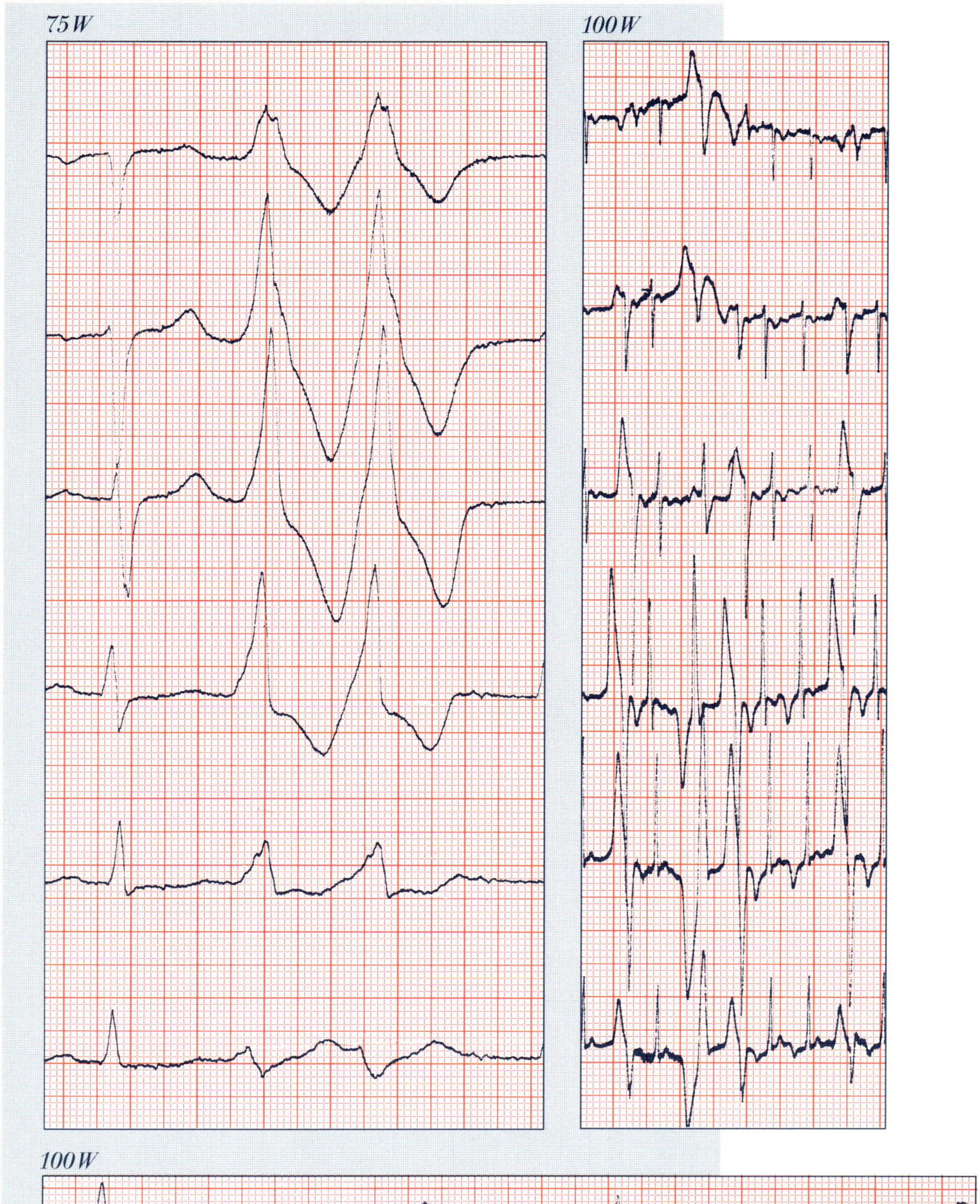

46-year-old patient without any structural heart disease, normal angiographic finding. Exercise testing shows new right bundle branch block (RBBB). No changes in ST segment in

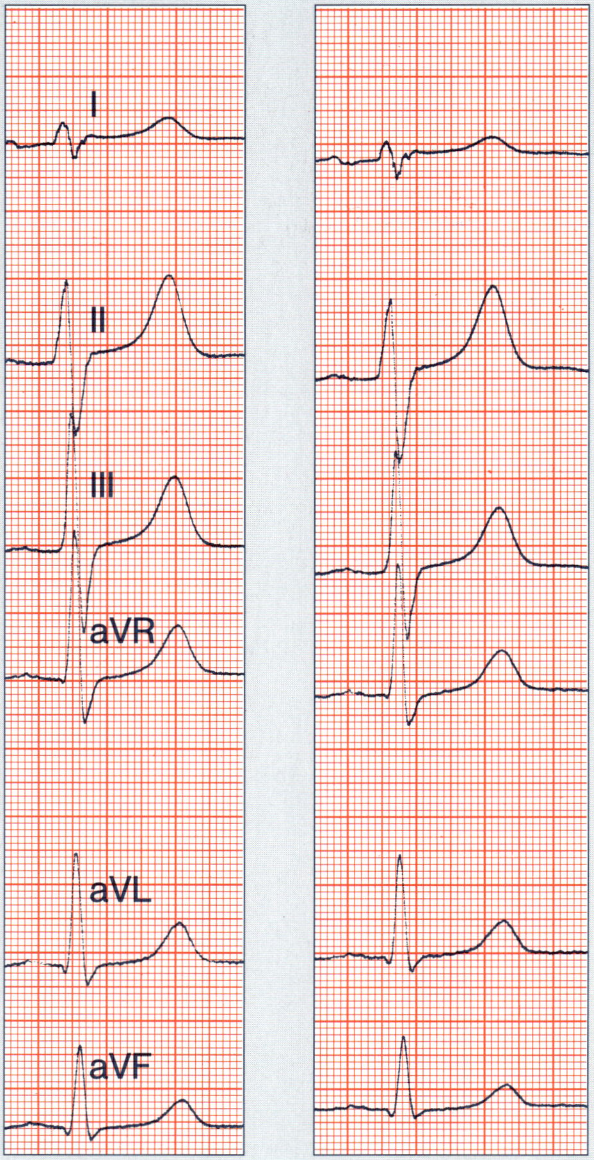

Rest

V_1-V_3 are only due to RBBB configuration. The coronary angiography was done as the patient wanted to continue and preserve his PPL (private pilot license).

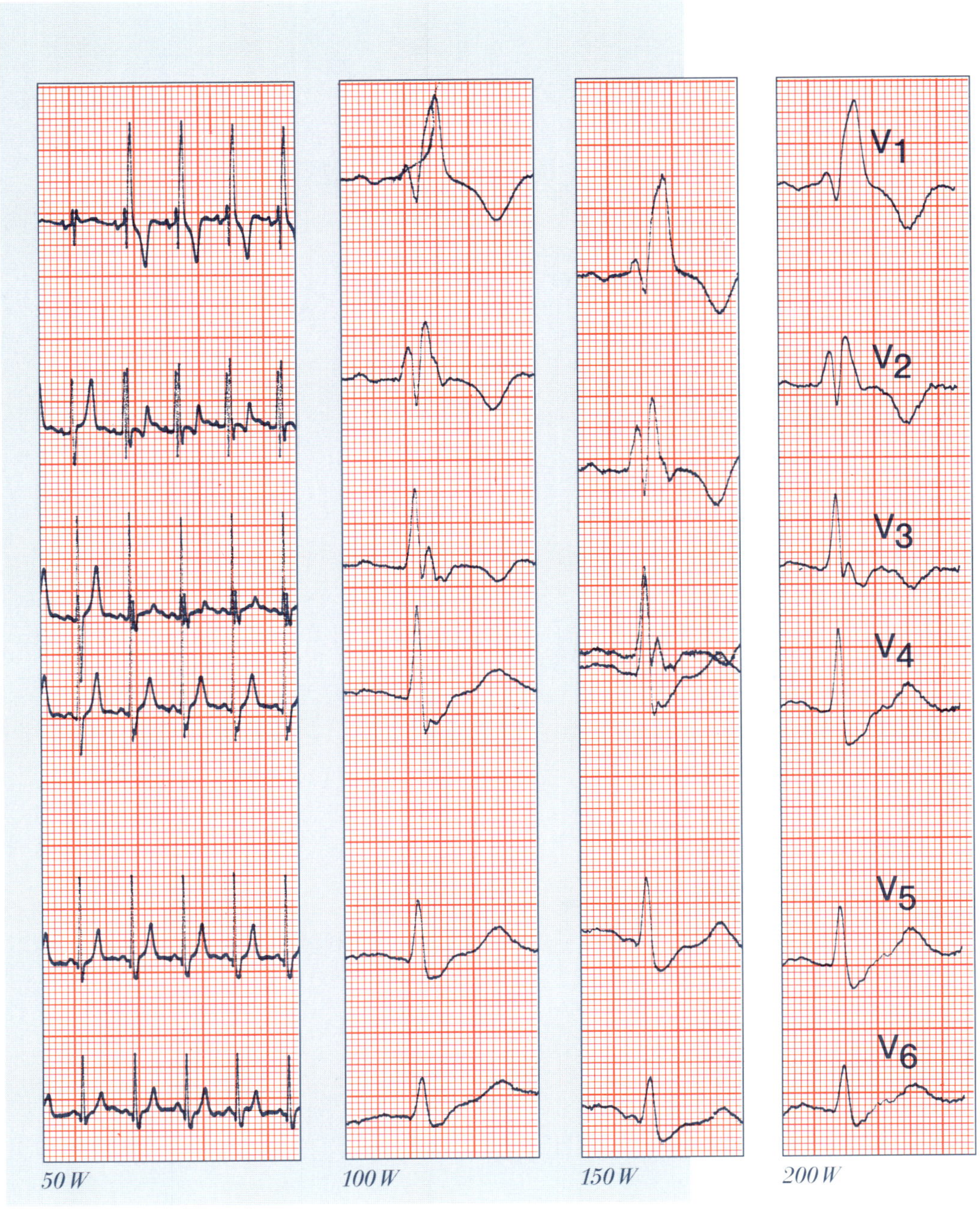

71-year-old patient with CAD and peripheral arterial occlusion. The ECG shows an old myocardial infarction, RBBB at rest and during exercise. During exercise testing there is ST segment depression in leads V_4-V_5 indicating exercise-induced

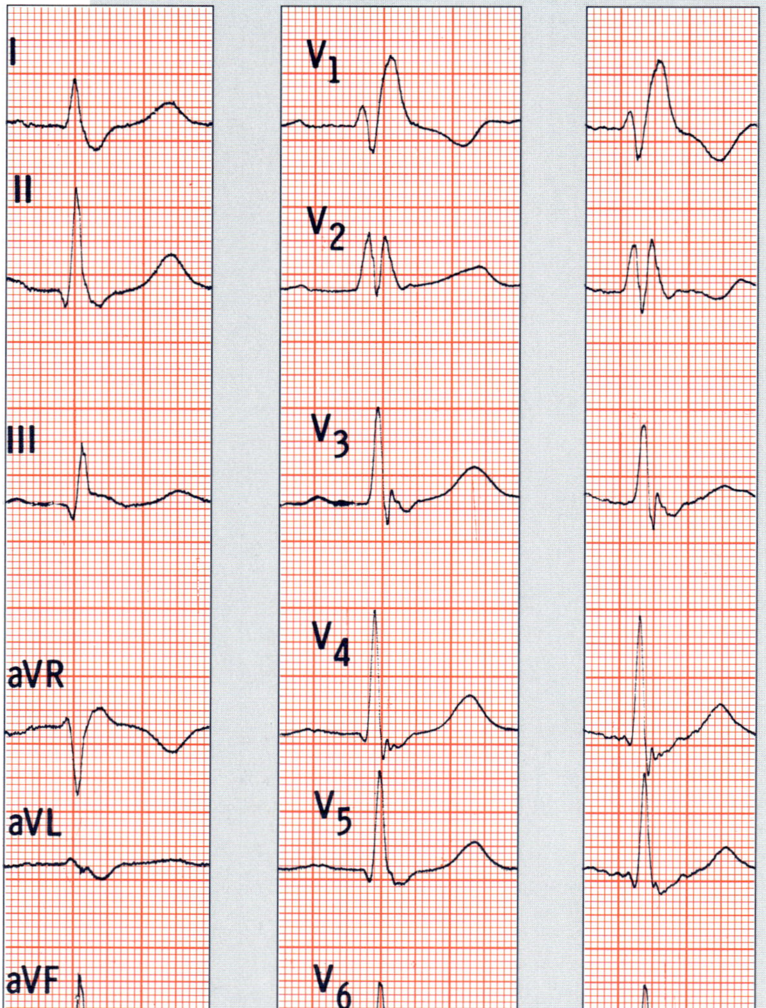

Rest *50W*

ischaemia. Thus, the changes in leads V_1-V_3 are due to RBBB, but changes in the left precordial leads V_4-V_6 are due to ischaemia.

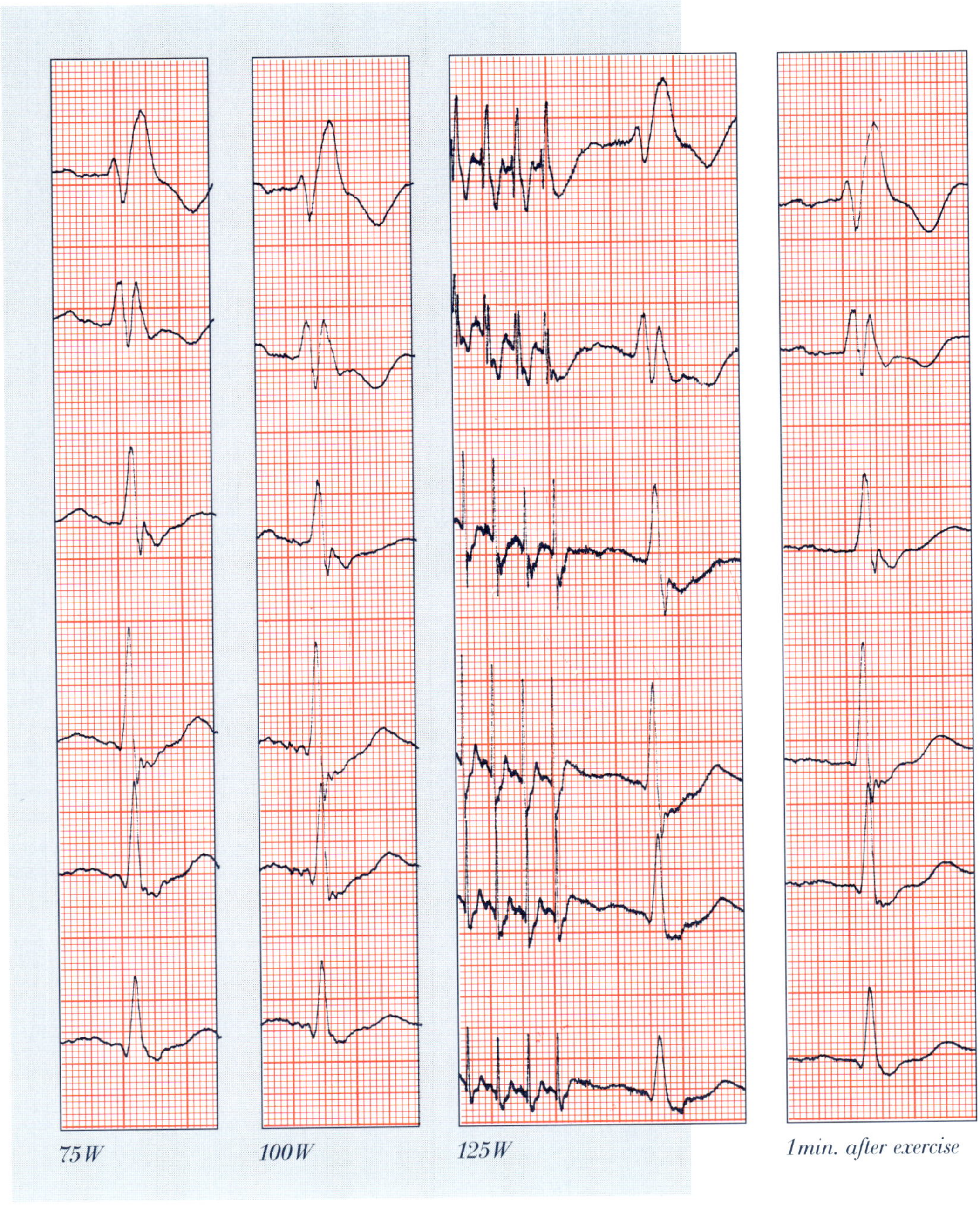

References

1. *Barold, S. S. (Hrsg.):* 12-Lead Electrocardiography. Cardiol. Clinics 5, Saunders, Philadelphia/London, 1987.
2. *Becker, H. J., G. Kober, M. Kaltenbach:* EKG - Repetitorium, Dtsch. Ärzteverlag, 1983, 3. Auflage.
3. *Bethge, K.-P.:* Langzeit-Elektrokardiographie bei Gesunden und Patienten mit koronarer Herzerkrankung. Springer-Verlag; Berlin, Heidelberg, New York, 1982.
4. *Börger, H. H.* (Bearbeitet von K. v. Olshausen): EKG – Information. Steinkopff Darmstadt, 1985, 5. Auflage.
5. *Chung, E. K.:* Ambulatory electro cardiography. Holter monitor electrocardiography. Springer-Verlag; New York, Heidelberg, Berlin, 1979.
6. *Csapo, G., D. Kalusche:* Konventionelle und intrakardiale Elektrokardiography. Cardiovascularia CIBA, CIBA-Geigy, Wehr, 1989, 2. Auflage.
7. *Dunn, M. I., B. S. Lipman, E. Massie:* Clinical Electrocardiography. Chicago, Year Book Publisher, 1989, 8th edition.
8. *Fish, C.:* Electrocardiography of arrhythmias, Philadelphia, Lea & Febinger, 1990.
9. *Fletscher, G. F.:* Dynamic electrocardiographic recording, Futura Publishing Company; Mount Kisco, New York, 1979.
10. *Goldman, M. J.:* Principles of Clinical Elektrocardiography, 11th edition, Lange, Los Altos, 1982.
11. *Heinecker, R.:* EKG in Praxis und Klinik, Thieme, Stuttgart, 1986, 12. Auflage.
12. *Höpp, H. W., A. Osterspey:* Langzeit-Elektrokardiographie, Kardiol. Diagnostik, Boehringer Mannheim, 1988, 2. Auflage.
13. *Josephson, M. E., S. F. Seides:* Clinical cardiac electrophysiology. Techniques and interpretations, Lea & Febinger, Philadelphia, 1979.
14. *Jeliffe, Roger W.:* Fundamentals of electrocardiography, New York, Springer-Verlag, 1990.
15. *Kennedy, H. L.:* Ambulatory electrocardiography including Holter recording technology, Lea & Febinger, Philadelphia, 1981.
16. *Klinke, R.:* Das Elektrokardiogramm, Thieme, Stuttgart, 1987, 5. Auflage.
17. *Kühn, P.:* EKG Fortbildung, Boehringer Mannheim, 1988.
18. *Lang, E.:* Kleines EKG-Seminar, Perimed Fachbuch Verlag, Erlangen, 1984, 8. Auflage.
19. *Lüderitz, B. (Hrsg.):* Herzrhythmusstörungen, Handbuch der Inneren Medizin, Band IX: Herz und Kreislauf, Springer; Berlin, Heidelberg, New York, 1983, 5. Auflage.
20. *Marriott, H. J. L.:* Practical Electrocardiography, Williams & Wilkins, Baltimore, 1988, 8th edition.
21. *Meinertz, T., M. Zehender, S. Hohnloser, A. Geibel:* Atlas der Langzeit-Elektrokardiographie, Fischer, Stuttgart, 1990.
22. *Mengden, H. J. v. (Hrsg.):* Vom EKG zur Diagnose, Thieme, Stuttgart, 1983.
23. *Mengden, H. J. v. (Hrsg.):* EKG-Diagnostik, Boehringer Mannheim, Reihe kardiologische Diagnostik, (1991) im Druck.
24. *Nusser, E., G. Trieb, A. Weidner:* Differentialdiagnostik des EKG, Schattauer, Stuttgart, New York, 1981, 2. Auflage.
25. *Roelandt. J. and P. G. Hugenholtz (Eds.):* Long-term ambulatory electrocardiography. Developments in cardiovascular medicine, Vol. 20. Martinus Nijhoff Publishers; The Hague, Boston, London, 1982.
26. *Sandoe, E., B. Sigurd:* Arrhythmia, Fachmed AG, St. Gallen, 1984.
27. *Schamroth, L.:* The disorders of cardiac rhythm (I und II): Blackwell, Oxford, 1980, 2. Auflage.
28. *Schamroth, L.:* The 12 lead elektrocardiogram, Boston, Blackwell Scientific, 1989.

29. *Seipel, L.:* Klinische Elektrophysiologie des Herzens. Thieme, Stuttgart, 1987, 2. Auflage.

30. *So, C. S.:* EKG-Schnellkurs, (Kardiologie Schwarz Pharma), Echo Verlags AG, Köln, 1989,

31. *So, C. S.:* Elektrokardiographie. Atlas und Auswertung, U & S., München, 1980, 2. Auflage.

32. *Stern. S.:* Ambulatory ECG monitoring. Year Book Medical Publishers; Chicago, London, 1978.

33. *Vlay, S.:* Manual of cardiac arrhythmias Liitle, Brown, Comp., Boston, Toronto, 1988.

34. *Wellens, H. J. J., H. E. Kulbertus (Eds.):* What's new in elektrocardiography? Martinus Nijhoff Publishers. The Hague, Boston, London, 1981.

35. *Wenger, N. K., M. B. Mock, I. Ringquist:* Ambulatory electrocardiographic recording. Year Book Medical Publishers; Chicago, London, 1981.

Literature referring to "Ergometry"

1. *American College of Sports Medicine:* Giudelines for exercise testing and prescription. Lea & Febinger, Philadelphia, 1986.
2. *Anlauf, M., K. D. Bock (Hrsg.):* Blutdruck unter körperlicher Belastung. Steinkopf, Darmstadt, 1984.
3. *Astrand, P.-O., K. Rodahl:* Textbook of work physiology. McGraw Hill, New York, 1977.
4. *Bachl, N., T. Graham, H. Löllgen (Eds.):* Advances in Ergometry. Springer, Heidelberg, New York, 1991.
5. *Cohn, J. N. (Eds.):* Quantitative exercise testing for the cardiac patient: The value of monitoring gas exchange. Circulation II, 76, 1987, Suppl. 6.
6. *Ellestad, M. H.:* Stress testing. 3. Aufl. Davis Comp., Philadelphia, 1986.
7. *Fardy, P. S., F. G. Yanowitz, P. K. Wilson:* Cardiac Rehabilitation, Adult Fitnes, and Exercise Testing. Lea & Febinger, Philadelphia, 1988.
8. *Fletscher, G. F., V. F. Froehlicher, H. Hartley, W. L. Haskell, M. L. Pollock:* Exercise standards. A statement for health professionals from the American Heart Association. Circulation 82, 1990, 2286-2322.
9. *Franklin, B. A., S. Gordon, G. C. Timmis:* Exercise in modern medicine. Williams and Wilkins, Baltimore, 1989.
10. *Franz, I.-W. (Hrsg.):* Belastungsblutdruck bei Hochdruckkranken. Springer Berlin, Heidelberg, New York, 1981.
11. *Froehlicher, V. F.:* Exercise and the heart. 2. Aufl. Year Book, Chicago, 1987.
12. *Hirzel, H. O.:* Ergometrische Belastung in der invasiven Diagnostik der koronaren Herzkrankheit. Thieme Copythek, Stuttgart, 1983.
13. *Hollmann, W., T. Hettinger:* Sportmedizin - Arbeits- und Trainingsgrundlagen. Schattauer, Stuttgart, 3. Auflage, 1990.
14. *Jones, N. L.:* Clinical Exercise Testing, 3. Auflage. Saunders, Philadelphia, 1988.
15. *Karpman, V. L.:* Cardiovascular System and Physical Exercise, CRC Press, 1987, Boca Raton, Florida.
16. *Leff, A. R.:* Cardiopulmonary Exercise Testing. Grune & Stratton, Orlando, New York, 1986.
17. *Lejemtel, T. H., D. Mancini, D. Gumbardo, B. Chadwick:* Pitfalls and limitations of maximal oxygen uptake as an index of cardiovascular functional capacity in patients with chronic heart failure. Heart Failure 1, 1985: 112-124.
18. *Lentner, C.:* Geigy Scientific Tables, **5**, Heart and Circulation, Basel, 1990, 8. Auflage.
19. *Löllgen, H., H. Mellerowicz:* Progress in ergometry, quality control and test criteria. Springer, Heidelberg, 1984.
20. *Löllgen, H., H.-V. Ulmer:* Ergometrie, Empfehlungen zur Durchführung und Bewertung ergometrischer Untersuchungen. Klin. Wschr. **63**, 1985: 651-677.
21. *Löllgen, H., H. Wollschläger, Y. Samstag, H. Just:* Belastungsdyspnoe bei Herz-Kreislauf-Erkrankungen - Übersicht und Probleme. In: Wylicil, P., W. Schale (Hrsg.): Belastungsdyspnoe bei Herz-Kreislauf-Erkrankungen. München, Gedon und Reuss, 1987, p. 51-74.
22. *Löllgen, H., H.-V. Ulmer, P. Crean (Hrsg.):* Recommendations and standard guidelines for ergometry. Europ. Heart J., Suppl. K., Nov. 1988, **9**: 1-37.
23. *Löllgen, H.:* Kardiopulmonale Funktionsdiagnostik, 2. Auflage. Doc. Geigy/Editio Ciba Wehr, 1990.
24. *McArdle, W. D., F. I. Katch, V. L. Katch:* Exercise Physiology, 2nd edition, Lea & Febinger, Philadelphia, 1985.
25. *McDougall, J. D., H. A. Wenger, H. J. Green:* Physiological Testing of the Elite Athlete. Mouvement Publications, Ithaca, NY, 1982.
26. *Mellerowicz, H., I.-W. Franz:* Standardisierung, Kalibrierung und Methodik in der Ergometrie. Perimed, Erlangen, 1983.
27. *Myers, J., V. F. Froehlicher*: Optimizing the exercise test for pharmacological investigations. Circulation **82**, 1990: 1839-1845.

28. *Naughton, J:* Exercise Testing: Physiological, Biomechanical and Clinical Principles. Futura Publishing Comp., New York, 1988.
29. *Packer, M.:* How should we judge the efficacy of drug therapy in patients with chronic congestive heart failure? The insights of six blind men. J. Am. Coll. Cardiol. **9**, 1987: 433-438.
30. *Pfisterer, M. E.:* Nuklearmedizinische Herzdiagnostik. Springer, Berlin, Heidelberg, New York, 1982.
31. *Reindell, H. und Mitarb.:* Funktionsdiagnostik des gesunden und kranken Herzens. Thieme, Stuttgart, 1988.
32. *Rost, R., W. Hollmann:* Belastungsuntersuchungen in der Praxis. Thieme, Stuttgart, 1982.
33. *Schlant, R. C., C. G. Blomquist, R. O. Brandenburg, R. DeBusk, M. H. Ellestad, G. F. Fletcher, V. F. Jr. Froehlicher, R. J. Hall, B. D. Mc.Callister, P. L. McHenry, T. J. Ryan, L. T. Sheffield:* Special report. Guidelines for exercise testing. A report of the Joint American College of Cardiology /American Heart Association Task Force on Assessment of Cardio-vascular Procedures (Subcommittee on Exercise Testing), Circulation **74**, 1986: 653 A-667 A.
34. *Schlant, R. C., G. C. Friesinger II, J. L. Leonhard:* Clinical competence in exercise testing. Circulation **82**, 1990: 1884-1888.
35. *Skinner, J. S:* Exercise testing and exercise prescription for special cases. Lea & Febinger, Philadelphia, 1987.
36. *Teitz, C. C. (Hrsg.):* Scientific foundations of sports medicine. B. C. Decker, Toronto, 1989.
37. *Wasserman, K.:* New concepts in assessing cardiovascular function. Circulation 78, 1988: 1060-1071.
38. *Wasserman, K., J. E. Hansen, D. Y. Sue, B. J. Whipp:* Principles of exercise testing and interpretation. Lea & Febinger, Philadelphia, 1987.
39. *Wasserman, K. (Eds.):* Measures of functional capacity in patients with heart failure. Circulation 81, 1990, Suppl. II.
40. *Weber, K. T., J. S. Janicki:* Cardiopulmonary exercise testing. Saunders, Philadelphia, 1986.
41. *Wylicil, P., W. Schale:* Belastungsdyspnoe bei Herz-Kreislauf-Erkrankungen. Gedon & Reuss, 1987.